GET REAL
ABOUT WEIGHT LOSS

By

Anu Morgan

Personal Development Publishing

Publisher's Cataloging-in-Publication Data
    Morgan, Anu.
        Get real about weight loss / by Anu Morgan. -- 1st ed.
          p. cm.
        Includes bibliographical references and index.
        LCCN 2009934082
        ISBN-13: 978-0-9755-9142-0 (pbk.)
        ISBN-10: 0-9755-9142-8 (pbk.)
        1. Reducing diets. 2. Reducing exercises.
        I. Title.
        RM222.2.M67 2009   613.2'5
                                 QBI09-600134

DEDICATION

Thanks to my husband, Scott. I could not have made this book happen without your help.

ACKNOWLEDGEMENTS

This book was made possible with the help of several people. Thanks to you all.

Thank you to Angel Guerrero for all of your hard work during the photo shoots. You are a great photographer! Thanks also to Alma Guerrero for doing the makeup for the exercise shoot and to Darcie Teasley for the cover shoot makeup and for making me look as good as possible. Thank you to Dennis Clendennen for doing such a great job on my hair during the cover shoot and making it work under the humid conditions. Thank you to John Michael Carlton for modeling with me in the exercise demonstration photos. Finally, thank you to Lily Pham for all of your administrative help in getting the book created. I appreciate you all!

TABLE OF CONTENTS

PREFACE

I've written this book because I genuinely want to help everyone who struggles to lose weight. Working as a personal trainer for ten years I have come in contact with so many people who all had one thing in common – an inability to lose weight and keep it off. Struggling with your weight is frustrating, hopeless, and discouraging, yet totally unnecessary. Weight loss and better physical health are attainable for everyone, and I want this book to give you the knowledge and tools necessary to make it happen for you!

Part One –

Setting the Stage

Chapter 1

Getting Started

There are now and always have been diet and exercise programs that promise easy success. Most people with a weight problem have tried many of these quick-fix solutions only to be disappointed with their lack of weight loss success. And the big question remains, "How am I ever going to lose this weight and keep it off?"

Well, I am here to help you finally solve the mystery. In this book, I am going to show you a simple yet incredibly effective approach to achieving weight loss. We will look at all the aspects of exercise and nutrition and give you a step-by-step plan to make it happen!

Now you may be asking yourself, "How is this approach going to be any different from all the others?" The answer is simple: it is a real life approach with real work involved.

You will get neither empty promises nor unrealistic advice. What you will get is a detailed, step-by-step, no-nonsense plan to lose weight and maintain that weight loss.

I am not going to bash the countless fad diets like Atkins, South Beach, or even the grapefruit diet. As you will find while reading the chapter on nutrition, all of these plans contain some elements that can help you lose weight, at least temporarily. But our goal is not just to lose weight but to keep it off **permanently**. You are about to finally learn exactly how to accomplish that. Let's summarize what we are going to go over.

Exercise Plan

The chapters on exercise will clearly lay out exactly the types and amount of exercise that you need to do. Yes, you read that correctly, there is exercise involved in this program. And believe me, you will want to exercise! Why? Because it takes a 3,500-calorie deficit to lose one pound! If you rely solely on your diet to create that deficit, it will take much, much longer. That is why you must also BURN OFF some calories. I know you want to get your results sooner rather than later and exercise can dramatically speed the process. Even more importantly, exercise is one of the key elements to maintaining your weight loss.

Diet Plan

The chapters on nutrition will first teach you the basics about carbohydrates, proteins, and fats. And then you will learn how to eat these foods in an effective way to help you lose weight. I will also provide you with a restaurant guide and help you learn how to make smart choices when dining out.

Potential Roadblocks

One of the main downfalls of many weight loss plans is their failure to recognize the real life limitations that frequently prevent people from achieving their desired weight loss. We are going to tackle these potential limitations head-on right from the start. It is important to recognize which of these roadblocks may apply to you so you can realistically deal with them from the outset and not let them hinder your efforts.

Potential Roadblock #1
Lack of Motivation

The biggest challenge for many is getting truly motivated. This is a subjective factor that can come and go in waves and either help you towards your goals or completely undermine your efforts. So you need to figure out how to keep yourself motivated, using this positive energy to help propel you towards your goal. I will help you with this in chapter 2, "Implementing the Plan."

Keep in mind that your desire can take you a long way in achieving success. As the old adage goes, "If you want something bad enough, you can get it." So if you truly want to lose weight and get in shape, my question for you is how bad do you want it? If it is very important to you it will be a priority and you will stay on course. If your desire wavers, then let me tell you right now – your likelihood of success will drop drastically. If you really, truly want to lose the weight, then that desire is what will get you through those tough times when you just don't feel like doing the work.

Potential Roadblock #2
Lack of Time

Another common roadblock is the lack of time. People are always saying how they don't have time to eat so they have to "eat on the run" and consequently they make very unhealthy choices. People often make a similar excuse about not having the time to exercise.

I know that many Americans lead busy, hectic lives. Yet some still manage to exercise regularly while working full-time jobs, raising children, and maintaining a home. Now I know that some people's circumstances really do make weight loss more challenging, but if you are truly motivated to finally stop making excuses and make your health a priority, then this plan can still be incorporated into your busy life and you still can lose the weight.

Potential Roadblock #3
Lack of Knowledge

A third possible roadblock is a lack of knowledge of exactly how to best go about losing the weight. You cannot succeed without the proper tools. This book is going to take care of the unknown and show you exactly how to use proper nutrition and exercise to help you reach your goals.

Potential Roadblock #4
Lack of Planning

Another potential obstacle is a lack of planning. For example, you wouldn't go into a test on exam day without having studied and expect to get an A. In the same way, you cannot go into a busy workday without having planned what and when you're going to eat, and when you plan to exercise. I'm not saying there has to be a rigid schedule in place every day, but you will need to do some planning and prioritizing to incorporate healthy eating and exercise into your day. This might seem like a lot of extra work initially, but after you get used to it you will find yourself automatically making healthier choices.

Potential Roadblock #5
Lack of Accountability

This one is a huge difference maker, yet it is often overlooked. Many people try to lose weight on their own and, while it is possible to do so, it sure is a lot tougher. It is very easy for people to get sidetracked, discouraged, and ready to throw in the towel if they do not have someone supportive to report to.

This is where a personal trainer can be very useful. As a personal trainer for over a decade I can tell you that one of the biggest benefits that my clients get is the feeling of accountability for sticking with the program. A personal trainer can help you be accountable for the amount of exercise you are doing and (if the trainer is knowledgeable on nutrition) for how well you are sticking to your diet.

If you feel like a personal trainer is out of your reach financially but you recognize how crucial accountability is going to be, you should really try out www.GetRealZone.com, my membership website. It can provide you with an economical version of accountability and support, with the convenience of an online format. Since I offer a free trial membership, you have nothing to lose, so go join now and get involved in the community. The members are people just like you who are working on becoming the fit person they have always wanted to be. There is just no substitute for having the support of people experiencing what you are experiencing, so give it a try now.

Chapter 2

Implement the Plan

The key to your success will be creating a plan and following it. Many people frequently think of how badly they want and need to lose weight, but very few ever create a specific plan of how to do it and then, more importantly, follow that plan. Weight loss doesn't just happen, it requires some thinking and planning. If you want to succeed, you must treat your weight loss project the way you would an important work project – by giving it attention, effort, and time. It is time to forget your old ways and tackle your weight loss with a new, fresh approach.

You are reading this book because you are looking for a solution to your problem. You have probably tried other plans in the past and did not get the results you wanted, or perhaps you lost weight but you did not keep it off. Let's examine why this may have happened by reviewing some of the most common diets and weight loss plans. It is important to identify your past pitfalls to avoid making the same mistakes this time around.

Low Carb Diets

You might be one of the many people who were on the Atkins diet for awhile. Many people (especially women) feel very deprived on this diet because of the extreme lack of carbohydrates. It can cause you to feel lethargic, irritable, to have difficulty focusing, or simply to have cravings for what you can't have. With such strong feelings of deprivation it is easy to understand why you might not succeed and how you could conclude that this particular diet is not for you.

Some people try the Atkins diet and love it, successfully losing weight. But then, as soon as they get off the diet and follow a more normal eating pattern (including more carbohydrates), the weight begins to creep back on.

You might also have tried the South Beach diet. It similarly restricts carbohydrate intake resulting in many of its dieters having the same experiences as the Atkins' dieters – feeling lethargic, irritable, and deprived.

Weight Loss Centers

You might also have tried something that promised a more systematic approach, such as

Weight Watchers. Weight Watchers is really more of a program than a diet because it is geared more towards teaching people how to eat.

In other words, Weight Watchers tells you specifically what and how much you should consume. The amount of food or calorie consumption is increased when you incorporate exercise into your life. The program offers a good overall structure, yet it still does not work for many. Why? Because it involves a lot of counting of calories, fat, and fiber. For most people the counting becomes somewhat overwhelming and takes the pleasure out of eating. It is just not enjoyable to get bogged down in the counting of your food. So for many people Weight Watchers is just not a realistic long-term solution.

You might also have tried other programs, like Quick Weight Loss Centers. Before I became a personal trainer I worked as a weight loss counselor for Quick Weight Loss, so I am very familiar with their program and the typical results. Like Weight Watchers, many of their clients do get positive results initially, only to have difficulty maintaining their weight loss after they get off the plan and go out on their own.

Most of these program-type solutions will require you to purchase their food products in order to follow their diet program. Since the program is structured in a way that makes it nearly impossible for you to follow the plan without purchasing their relatively expensive food, you become somewhat dependent on the program to maintain your weight loss. Obviously, this is a major disadvantage if your ultimate goal is to lose weight and permanently keep it off on your own.

Your Personalized Weight Loss Plan

Different approaches work for different people, but what works for everyone is a **personalized plan**! What do you need to know in order to create your own personalized plan? Very simply, you need to know yourself and analyze your needs.

For example, if you know that you dislike exercise and in the past have made a lot of excuses to avoid or put off exercising, then your personalized plan needs to include a way to make yourself accountable. Let's take a closer look at how to create your personalized plan. As I mentioned earlier, you will need to eat healthy and exercise to succeed. So we need to fill in all the gaps of how we can make that happen.

First, you will have to make the time to go to the grocery store on a regular and consistent basis. Having the proper foods in your refrigerator and pantry are a must so that you will be able to follow the healthy eating plan. So if you already see this as a problem, tackle it before moving on. Perhaps you can adjust your schedule and get your spouse to watch the kids in the evening while you go to the store to stock up. Maybe your busy work schedule doesn't leave you with much free time during the week, so you allot some time on the weekend for the grocery shopping. Whatever your limitations, you must find a way around them.

Next, you will have to exercise. The type and amount of exercise will vary a great deal based on your current level of fitness and your personal goals. We will discuss your particular exercise regimen in the exercise section of this book, but the point is you will need to find some time for it. If you currently feel you have no time to spare, then you need to assess your current schedule and decide how you will open up some time for exercise. The good news is that once you get started exercising you will be amazed at the increased level of energy you will have. The time you make for exercise will more than pay for itself in increased energy and self-esteem, I promise.

Now that we have established the importance of getting the right foods and making the time to exercise, we need to talk about cooking. You will find it much easier to consistently eat healthier if you make some of your meals at home. I'm not saying you can't eat out anymore and I'll actually give you some great tips on how to eat healthy while eating out in Chapter 10, "Restaurant Guide and Shopping Do's and Don'ts." But for now, we need to decide when you will prepare your meals.

If your weekdays are super hectic, then it is probably a good idea to do some cooking on the weekends in large quantities so you can have meals during the week that are already prepared. Yes, this does take planning and work, but it can really pay major dividends in the form of quick and easy healthy meals.

Now if you are thinking, there is no way I'm going to cook or you just flat don't know how to cook, there are still options for you. You can go through a food service in which they prepare meals according to your dietary needs, and some even deliver the food to you. Could that be any easier? In Houston, where I live, one such service is Diet Gourmet. While these services are not cheap, if you already eat most of your meals out then the prices are pretty comparable to what you are probably already paying.

Yet another option would be to buy pre-prepared food that many gourmet grocery stores now offer (for example, Whole Foods). Keep in mind though that all natural and/or organic foods don't necessarily equate low-calorie and low-fat foods. But, after reading about nutrition in this book you will be able to make healthy choices that are conducive to your weight loss goal.

Now that the major bases are covered, let's take a look at a sample plan. As an example, we'll use Cynthia, a married mother of three children, ages 4, 7, and 9. Cynthia has a busy work schedule as a partner at a large accounting firm, on top of being primarily responsible for the kids and maintaining the house. She has a part-time nanny to help some with the kids, but Cynthia does nearly all the cooking and shopping for the family. Here is the personalized plan she came up with:

Cynthia's Personalized Plan

Grocery Shopping

Since I don't want the kids distracting me while I am shopping, I will need to do the shopping either on Friday evening after work or sometime on the weekends. My husband can watch the kids while I am doing the shopping.

Cooking

Since I usually need to work late on Mondays and Wednesdays I will plan ahead so no cooking will be required. I will cook dinner for the family on Tuesday and Thursday night, and then on the weekends I will cook large quantities so that there are leftovers for extra nights, as well as to give me healthy meals to take for lunches.

Eating Out

If I am picking, I will chose restaurants that have a reasonable amount of healthy options. If the circumstances require me to go somewhere that doesn't have many healthy options, I will order modifications to my meal (like no oil, no butter) to make it healthier.

Exercise

Monday and Wednesday evenings are out for exercise because of work. I will work out on Tuesday and Thursday mornings, before I go to the office. I will also exercise on Saturday morning. For now, I will do a home-based workout with dumbbells and my treadmill, but I plan on joining a gym next month.

<u>Accountability</u>

Since I have had difficulty in the past staying on track I will get a free trial membership to Anu's GetRealZone.com. This will allow me to keep an online journal and the supportive GetRealZone community will help me create some accountability.

Cynthia commits to review her personalized plan once a week so she can see if she is sticking with her plan. As circumstances change she can modify her plan to better fit her life but the plan will help her to regularly stay on track.

Changes she might consider in the future could include:

- hire a cook to prepare meals for the family
- get food from a food service with her dietary specifications
- have the nanny put in some extra hours so Cynthia has more time for the food preparation
- exercise with her spouse or a friend to help motivate each other

- get the class schedule from her gym and consider doing aerobics or other classes
- hire a personal trainer

These are just some ideas that may be applicable to you. The point is for you to really stop and think right now of the roadblocks you may face and find a way to overcome them. Have faith; others have been exactly where you are who successfully lost weight. So why not let it happen for you?

Chapter 3

Make the Commitment

So what does it take to truly commit to losing weight? It begins with a true desire. When you want something bad enough you will do whatever it takes. That means you need to be passionate about your new weight loss endeavor. When you feel enthusiastic about your goal, that passion will carry you through any minor obstacles or setbacks you may have. So let's consider a few questions to help you decide if you are really passionate about your goal and ready to make the commitment:

1. How badly do you want to lose weight?
2. What would it mean to you to reach your weight loss goal?
3. Are you willing to make sacrifices to meet your goals? What sacrifices?

4. Are you willing to modify your habits?
5. Are you prepared to put work into losing weight?
6. Are you ready to make weight loss one of your top priorities?
7. Are you doing this for yourself?
8. What will it mean to you if you don't succeed in losing weight?

If you haven't answered these questions, stop and take the time to do it. It will be worth your while.

Now let's review your answers. Your answers to numbers 1 and 2 should make it clear that you want to lose weight badly and it is a big deal to you. Such a big deal that it is frequently in the forefront of your thoughts.

Numbers 3 to 6, you should have answered with a definitive "YES!" If you thought "'maybe" then you need to reevaluate your desire. I have helped enough people lose weight that I know the commonalities shared by those who succeed. Universally, the people who lose weight do all the things that questions 3 to 6 ask of you.

Question number 7, whether you are doing this for yourself, is an important question. Your answer needs to be, undoubtedly yes. You will not succeed or do it with pleasure if you are not doing it for yourself. This is one of those rare times in life where it is all about YOU! Now is your opportunity to be selfish.

I can tell you right now, if the only reason you are doing this is to make someone else happy, don't even bother. You must want this for yourself if you are to succeed. Pleasing someone else is simply not strong enough motivation to keep you going when the going gets tough.

In addition to all the practical steps you will take in your weight loss journey, there are three additional steps you can take that will dramatically improve your chances of success. Those three steps are visualization, creating a support system, and rewarding yourself as you progress towards your goal.

Visualization

If you have never done any form of visualization before, the idea might seem far out and a little weird to you, but just hear me out.

Many professional athletes frequently use the power of visualization to improve their performance. The athlete will vividly imagine himself performing at a near perfect level over and over. Many well-documented studies have proven that visualization can dramatically improve athletic performance. The reason for this is simple: the mind has a very hard time distinguishing between an actual event and a vividly imagined event. The end result is that vividly imagined events can help you establish a routine or a habit in a much more effective and rapid fashion than if you only used actual experiences.

So how does this relate to you and your weight loss goal? Well, just like the athlete who pictures his muscles moving in the desired way to make a play, you too can picture yourself taking action that will help you attain your goals.

For example, let's say that your goal is to lose twenty pounds and one of the obstacles to achieving your goal is your habit of eating lunch with coworkers at a fast food restaurant where you always order a greasy burger and fries. You can use visualization to picture yourself going to that same restaurant, but instead of a burger and fries, ordering something healthy like a grilled chicken salad with fat-free dressing. If you picture this event over and over in your mind, when the time comes you will find it much easier to resist temptation. Why? Because your mind subconsciously believes that you have the habit of making a healthy choice in that situation. Try it and you will become a believer!

Let's look at another example of how visualization can be used to help you reach your goal. Sticking with the goal of a twenty-pound weight loss, you can use visualization to help that goal seem more attainable and real.

Here is what you do. First relax, close your eyes, and take a few calming deep breaths. Now imagine yourself putting on a pair of pants that are currently a bit snug. Now vividly picture those exact same pants, easily slipping on; in fact, they are really kind of loose on your waist and just hanging on your body. Those same pants that were too tight are now about two sizes too big for you! Really feel and experience the exhilaration and excitement of successfully transforming your body into what you want it to be.

Do this exercise for just a couple of minutes a day and you will really increase your level of motivation and you will almost magically begin to feel like your goal is very realistic and not so far-fetched. The thing is that your imagination and your subconscious are working all the time anyway. The question is whether you will take some control and let that imagination work for you, or if you will ignore it and allow it to work against you.

Imagine yourself achieving your goals and making your fantasy a reality!

Create a Support Network for Yourself

The second thing you can do to help yourself reach your goals is to create a solid support network. You need at least a few people who know what you are trying to achieve who can give you encouragement.

Who comprises your support team will be different for different people. If you are married, then hopefully your spouse will be on board with you and fully supportive of the things you will be doing to lose weight. Ideally, you could do this as a joint project with your spouse.

If you are single then the people you spend a lot of your time with will play a prominent role. For example, let's say you have a group of friends who like to go out to eat and drink a lot, then you will need to either avoid going out with them or see if they are receptive to places with healthier options. You might even try to get one of your friends to join you in your weight loss project. The best kind of support is someone who is experiencing exactly what you are experiencing, so a buddy who is also trying to lose weight can really be helpful.

Rewarding Yourself for Progress

Lastly, another key to improving your chances of success is the reward system. The idea is to provide yourself with positive reinforcement every time you reach a short term goal.

So if your main goal is to lose thirty pounds, it is a good idea to set a few mini-goals along the way. Let's say your first mini-goal is to lose 6 pounds in 4 weeks. Once you get there, you should do something for yourself that you normally would not do. It can be cheap or expensive, anything from your spouse giving you a night off and taking care of the kids to buying yourself a piece of jewelry.

You want to keep this process fun and motivating. Positive reinforcement is always a great thing and probably the best way to encourage similar positive behavior. After all, it has proven to be effective in the workplace. When employers acknowledge and reward the efforts of their employees, they benefit from improved productivity. So why not reward yourself to help keep the good results coming?

Chapter 4

Setting Goals

Before we get down to the details of exercise and diet, you need to first set some short term and long term goals. It would be helpful if you wrote them down so you can refer back to them.

This is where things get real and where you need to be realistic. You might have just a little weight to lose or a lot. Either way, this plan will work for you. But you need to start with realistic goals and expectations of yourself.

What Measurements Should My Goals Be Based On?

There are four different measurements that can be used to track your progress:

1. weight scale
2. body circumference measurements
3. body fat measurements
4. how your clothes fit

Weight Scale

First, let's discuss the one people are most familiar with, the weight scale. The scale is very helpful as a tracking tool if you are trying to lose a significant amount, say twenty pounds or more, but much less important if you are just trying to lose just a few pounds.

For someone trying to lose a minor amount of weight (five pounds or less) it is not worthwhile to obsess over the scale. Since our bodies are made up of approximately 65-75% water, fluctuations of a few pounds may not coincide with actual weight loss and may have more to do with increases or decreases in how much water your body is retaining. For a weight loss of just a few pounds you should use another measure to monitor your progress, like circumference measurements, which we will discuss below.

If you want to lose ten pounds or more, then the readings on the scale will be a quick and easy way for you to periodically track your progress. Taking body measurements is also recommended here as well, to get a thorough and complete picture of your progress, so let's discuss that now.

Body Circumference and Body Fat Measurements

The simplest way to do this is to get out an old-fashioned tape measure and check the circumference measurements on the key body areas you are concerned with, which may include:

- Chest
- Waist
- Stomach
- Hips
- Thigh
- Calf
- Bicep

For a handy form you can print out and use to periodically keep track of these measurements, visit GetRealZone.com/form1/.

If you really want an accurate measurement of your body composition then body fat analysis can also be done to evaluate your initial level and monitor your progress. Normally this would require the assistance of a personal trainer or other fitness professional.

Body fat is most often assessed using a device known as calipers. When doing this assessment, it is important that two variables remain constant. First, good quality calipers should be used, and second, the same individual should do the measurement each time so the room for error is minimized. Because the measurements are performed differently by different professionals, it is quite possible that two trainers could measure the same person and get significantly different measurements. If the same person does the measurement each time you will get an accurate indication of your actual progress.

Keep in mind, body fat readings have a few percent margin of error, but they give you a good relative indicator of your progress and help measure your improvement as your body fat decreases and your lean muscle mass increases. Since lean muscle weighs more than fat, this is very important to know so that you don't become overly dependent on just the weight scale.

Measuring Your Progress
By How Your Clothes Fit

The last is much less scientific but can be a very good indicator of how much progress you are making. You simply monitor your progress by how your clothes fit.

Although this kind of measurement produces no numerical value that you can record, it can nonetheless be a very helpful tool to check your progress. For example, if you find that your clothes begin to hang off of you and the skinny jeans that you haven't worn in years fit perfectly, then you can rest assured that you are making progress. This is true no matter what the scale says.

The scale can actually be misleading in some cases. As an example, let's take a person who wanted to lose ten pounds. She was relatively thin and had never exercised or lifted weights. When she begins lifting weights and exercising she will begin to gain lean muscle mass at the same time she is losing fat. Since muscle weighs more than fat, she may at first actually gain weight while she is getting trimmer and leaner. If she only pays attention to the scale she may get frustrated, believing she is not making any progress. But the clothes don't lie – if she drops from a size eight to a size four, I don't care what the scale says, she is going to get pretty excited!

Goal Setting Specifics

You may be asking, what is the point of all this goal setting? The objective is to keep you focused. On the road to weight loss, it is very easy to become frustrated or get sidetracked. If you have concrete goals you can refer back to them and they will help you stay focused on your objective. When you have that momentary feeling that the weight is just not coming off as fast as you want, you can look back at your starting point and see all the progress that you have made. This will re-inspire you to stick with the program.

So the next question is, what are realistic goals for you? This can be a tricky question. Everyone's body is different and everyone will have a different idea of what they want their body to look like.

Before we get into creating your specific goals, let's go over a few basic definitions that will help determine a healthy weight for you. A very basic way to determine what your target weight should be is your body mass index, or "BMI." This is the one a doctor might use to tell you what your ideal weight is. It is a mathematical equation that divides your weight by your height. To calculate BMI, the following equation is used:

$$BMI = \frac{\text{Bodyweight (in kilograms)}}{\text{Height (in meters)}^2}$$

The BMI (shown on the next page) has the following range to determine whether a person's weight is appropriate:

BMI less than 25	Normal weight
BMI of 25 – 29.9	Overweight
BMI of 30-39.9	Obese
BMI of 40 or more	Morbidly obese

As an example we'll use a man who is 5'10" and weighs 200 pounds. One pound equals 0.4536 kilograms and one inch equals 0.0254 meters, so converted to metric he weighs 91 kilograms and is 1.78 meters tall. Using the calculation, his BMI is 25.6, or "overweight," according to the BMI scale.

Before you get too obsessed with the BMI scale, just keep in mind it does not differentiate fat weight from muscle weight. And, what that means is, if you have a lot of muscle and are the same height as the next person who has more fat, your BMI would be higher. The example given above could be someone very out of shape with a 44-inch waist or it could be an NFL running back with only 6% body fat. The BMI scale is very simplistic and does not take into account body fat, age, or gender. Nonetheless, it is a good starting point to consider when deciding on your target weight.

Now let's consider some sample 30 Day Goals based on the total amount of weight you are trying to lose.

Lose 15 Pounds or Less

Since your body does not have that much fat, the rate at which the pounds come off will be a little slower for you than someone who has a lot of weight to lose. You can expect to lose between one and two pounds per week at the most. While there are ways to lose weight more quickly, these are generally unhealthy strategies that are not designed to help you keep the weight off. As far as inches are concerned, you can expect to drop 1-3 sizes depending on your muscle gains vs. fat loss, and your body type.

If you fall under this category a sample 30 Day Goal could be: *Lose 4-8 pounds in the first 30 days.*

Lose Between 15 and 30 Pounds

Since your body can afford to let go of more weight, it will come off a bit quicker. You will perhaps see more than 2 pounds per week for the first couple of weeks, and then you also can expect it to level off at one to two pounds per week. As far as inches are concerned, you can expect to lose several inches. If you fall under this category a sample 30 Day Goal could be: *Lose 8-10 pounds in the first 30 days.*

Lose 30 Pounds or More

For someone with thirty or more pounds to lose, you also can expect to lose two or more pounds a week initially, but your weight loss will remain accelerated beyond just the first couple of weeks. You can also expect to lose several inches.

If you fall under this category, a sample 30 Day Goal could be: Lose 15 pounds in the first 30 days.

After reading the sample goals, you should have a better idea of what is realistic for your body type. It should be obvious that you will not drop 15 pounds in the first month if overall you only have 20 pounds to lose. Also, keep in mind that the sample goals are only guidelines. It is up to you to create and write down your specific goals and exactly how you want your body to change.

In addition to the aesthetic goals we have discussed you can also set fitness goals. For example, if you have a difficult time jogging one mile, but would really like to see yourself improve, then why not aim to build up your endurance to three miles over the next several months. If you are able to use a cardio machine for only five minutes, then set a goal of adding one to two minutes each time you engage in cardiovascular exercise.

You can also set a strength goal. For example, if you are able to do a one-arm curl with a five pound dumbbell then try building up to a ten pound dumbbell. Believe me, when you start to challenge your body with fitness goals, you will see great aesthetic results that follow!

Part Two –

The Workout

Chapter 5

Cardiovascular Exercise

Finally, it is time to talk about exercise! In this chapter, we will discuss cardiovascular (or cardio) exercise, including how much and how often you should do it, as well as some creative ideas on how to keep it interesting and fun.

As the name suggests, cardiovascular exercise works the heart muscle. The more you work the heart through exercise, the stronger that muscle becomes. It is no different in its response to exercise than the other muscles in your body, such as your arms and legs.

While strengthening your heart is certainly reason enough to regularly do cardio, the primary benefit for weight loss purposes is that, properly done, cardio will help you burn a lot of calories! Isn't that a great reason to get off your butt? Remember, weight loss is not complicated.

When you consistently burn more calories than you consume you will lose weight. It is that simple.

Let's discuss some of the key elements about cardio, including the mode or type of cardio you should choose, the intensity of your cardio, and the frequency and duration of your cardio sessions.

What Type of Cardio Should You Do?

Choosing which type (or mode) of cardio to do is an important decision. Cardio can be anything from walking to rock climbing.

Start by considering what kinds of activities you like to do. Do you enjoy walking outside and getting fresh air, dancing to music, jogging in the park, rollerblading, doing aerobics, biking? If you select forms of cardio that you like you will be far more likely to continue doing it. By having several different modes of cardio that you rotate through you can prevent boredom and injury. Additionally, changing up the modes of cardio will help your body burn more calories. By not allowing your body to get overly acclimated to any single activity, your body will be continually challenged and you will maximize the amount of calories expended.

Here are a few different modes of cardio to jumpstart your imagination:

- Walking – briskly
- Jogging
- Biking
- Jumping rope
- Dancing – fast pace
- Aerobic classes
- Skiing
- Skating
- Rollerblading
- Swimming
- Hiking
- Elliptical trainer
- Step climber machine
- Rowing machine

And, don't forget about sports! If you enjoy them, it is a fabulous way to make your cardio enjoyable. The key is that the sport should involve a lot of constant movement, enabling your heart rate to stay elevated. For example, baseball, golf, and table tennis are not good choices because you spend too much time standing still. Here are some ideal sports for cardio:

- Tennis
- Racquetball
- Basketball
- Football
- Soccer
- Volleyball

- Hockey
- Track

How Intense Should Your Cardio Be?

Intensity refers to the level of difficulty of your cardio exercise. This factor is extremely important. You want to do your cardio at a very challenging level so that your heart rate will be sufficiently elevated to burn the maximum amount of calories you are capable of expending.

The duration or the time you exercise is also of great importance. There is a big difference between doing ten minutes versus 30 minutes of cardio. Lastly, the frequency or the number of times you exercise each week will greatly affect your success rate.

There are two common methods to evaluate how hard you should be working when you do your cardio. The first involves a calculation of your target heart rate range and then checking your heart rate while exercising to ensure that you are within that range. The second has a fancy name (the Borg Scale of Rate of Perceived Exertion) but is actually a lot simpler to apply and usually works quite well.

To do the heart rate range calculation you first subtract your age from 220. This serves as a handy estimate, but it should be noted that the maximum heart rate can vary a lot from person to person. When you have calculated your maximum heart rate, you then multiply that number by 65% for the low end of the range and 85% for the high end of the range.

Let's use a forty-year-old as an example and calculate his heart rate range:

220 - 40 = 180	Maximum heart rate
180 x .85 = 153	High end of range
180 x .65 = 117	Low end of range

This is the heart rate range within which most individuals should do their cardio. If you find that this range does not challenge you enough (for those in better cardiovascular health this may be the case) you can then exceed the recommended range and use the rate of perceived exertion (RPE) as your guide, which we will discuss below.

After you know your range, you then need to periodically measure your heart rate while exercising. You can take this measurement by placing your index and middle fingers on your jugular vein (located on the side of the neck) or your wrist (below the thumb). Feel the beats for 15 seconds and then multiply that number by four to get your current heart rate. If you don't like doing it manually you could also try a heart rate monitor that straps across your chest under your shirt. Note that while many cardio machines claim to measure your heart rate and they can be used to get a relative idea of how hard you are working, they are notoriously inaccurate when it comes to their actual readings.

The second (and simpler) method to monitor your intensity is by using the Borg Scale of Rate of Perceived Exertion (RPE). The original Borg scale has been simplified even further with a 1-1-10 range scale (see below).

Exertion Level	Borg	Description
1	6	no exertion
	7-8	extremely light
2	9-10	very light
3-4	11-12	light
5-6	13-14	somewhat hard
7-8	15-16	hard
8.5-9	17-18	very hard
9.5	19	extremely hard
10	20	maximum exertion

The American College of Sports Medicine (ACSM) says an exertion level of between 4 and 6 correlates to 60-85% of your maximum heart rate.

The advantage of the RPE scale is its simplicity. No complicated calculations or heart rate measurements are required. The disadvantage is that it is very subjective and thus, you might find yourself not working nearly as hard as you should. Let me clarify what is meant by working "somewhat hard." If you can easily hold a conversation while doing your cardio, then you are probably working "light" or "very light."

In order to determine what exertion level you should be working at, we need to first define your current fitness level as either beginner, intermediate, or advanced.

A beginner is someone who has never done any cardiovascular exercise or who has not done any cardio in the past six months or more. An intermediate is someone who does some form of cardiovascular exercise either occasionally (maybe twice a week) or inconsistently, but does not let more than a week or so pass between cardio sessions. Finally, the advanced person does some form of cardiovascular exercise consistently between four and six times per week. An advanced person is not necessarily an athlete, but is simply more consistent about cardio than the other groups.

The beginners should perform the majority of their cardio between a 4 and 5. Intermediates should be doing 5 to 6 and the advanced should be working between 5 and 9.5, with most of the session between 5 and 8 with short occasional intervals that go above 8.

The benefit to working at a higher RPE is that as you are working harder your heart is pumping faster and you are burning more calories. Of course, you should work in the ranges specified for your current fitness level. Trying to do too much too soon will cause you to overexert yourself, which can result in feeling "wiped out" and lead to a loss of motivation. Worse yet, you could suffer an injury and sidetrack your efforts for a period of time. So be patient with yourself; after a few weeks you will feel your endurance building up and you can then begin to increase the intensity.

Duration of Your Cardio Sessions

How long should your cardio sessions last? Ideally, 30 minutes is a goal you should work towards. If you are a beginner, initially you will not be able to go this long and that is fine. If at first you do five minutes, that's great, you have done the hardest part – you have gotten started!

The next day you can work on increasing to six minutes and by the next week you might be up to ten minutes. The key thing to remember is to keep your intensity between a 4 and 6 on the RPE scale. If you are an intermediate, you might come close to 30 minutes or you might even be able to do the full 30 minutes.

For the advanced, you should be able to do the full 30 minutes and then some. And if you feel like doing more than 30 minutes, go for it. It won't hurt you, it will only help. Remember that you can always exercise at a higher intensity level (for example, by using brief periods of high intensity intervals) and then the 30 minutes will be more than sufficient.

Just remember that you will have to find a balance for yourself for time management purposes. This balance will consist of your weight training workouts, your work schedule and availability, and how often you are doing cardio.

Frequency of Your Cardio Sessions

Ideally, you should do cardio five times per week. I know this might sound like a lot, but I can promise you that you will get your best results and will begin shedding pounds more rapidly if you do it this frequently. After you have reached your target weight you could scale this frequency back somewhat, but while you are trying to lose weight I really recommend five cardio sessions per week.

If your lifestyle and circumstances don't allow you to fit cardio in five times a week, at a minimum you should do three times per week.

Don't misunderstand what I am saying. I am not giving you an excuse or permission to do it less than five times per week. To get the best and most rapid results, I definitely recommend five times a week and if you cut back to three simply because you are being lazy, then you might want to refer back to Chapter 3 about making the commitment to yourself.

Additionally, you might have an off week here or there and that is okay. You don't have to be perfect; just do your best to consistently get in five sessions per week and you will really be impressed with the outcome. The fact that you are getting off your butt and moving regularly will start to make a big difference. The more consistent you are the faster you will see results.

For most people exercising five times a week seems like a lot. But our bodies were not created to be sedentary. For most people today it is becoming difficult to maintain a healthy weight. This is becoming especially true of the younger generation.

While diet certainly plays a role, the primary reason for this is that we are simply not moving enough. Some of you who live in large cities like New York tend to walk more and drive less and that is great. But for most Americans, the majority of their walking is done going to and from their cars.

This is one of the differences that cause Europeans to not be as overweight as Americans. They walk a lot more on a daily basis. You might remember the book, *French Women Don't Get Fat*. The major premise was that, while the French are able to eat high fat foods like cheese and chocolate along with wine, they don't get fat because their portion sizes are much smaller than typical American portions. While it is true that the French (along with other Europeans) do eat smaller portions than Americans, that is only part of the equation. The other part is that extensive walking is a routine part of most Europeans' daily lives.

So the next time you feel exercising five times a week is too much, remember that it is natural for your body to keep moving. We were not designed to be sedentary.

Lastly, if going to the gym and doing the same old routine is getting mundane, then find some variety and enjoyment in your exercise regimen. You can achieve this through changing things up and trying some of the examples listed earlier in this chapter. Get a workout partner, hire a personal trainer, or jog on an outdoor trail. If you have been cooped up all winter, when the spring and summer roll around you can implement more outdoor activities, such as biking, swimming, or tennis. When you start to feel bored with it, get creative!

Choosing a Gym or Personal Trainer

Since many people will choose to join a health club so that they have access to cardio and other fitness equipment, let's briefly discuss how you should select a gym. First, you want to pick a gym that you are comfortable with. Just base this on how you feel about it when you visit. If you are a beginner and you visit a gym that makes you uncomfortable because it is filled with 300 pound bodybuilders then that is probably not the right gym for you.

Second, you want to pick a gym that has a convenient location. Decide whether it would be more convenient to have a gym that is closer to your home or work and then look in that area. You will find it much easier to get there on a regular basis if it is conveniently located!

Another issue we should address is hiring a personal trainer. A lot of beginners choose to do this and, while not absolutely necessary, it can be very helpful in staying focused and reaching your goals. When hiring a personal trainer you again need to go with your instincts about who you feel comfortable with. Some factors you might consider include gender, age, fitness level, and personality. You want to make sure the trainer is experienced and, preferably, has a college degree in a fitness-related field and a nationally accredited certification such as ACE

(American Council on Exercise) or ACSM (American College of Sports Medicine).

Chapter 6

Weight Training Exercise

Along with the cardiovascular exercise, you will need to incorporate weight training if you are serious about losing weight and keeping it off. And, yes, this applies to both men and women.

Women Need Weight Training Too

Many women have the completely unfounded misconception that if they lift weights they will become bulky and muscular. This is completely false. I have been training women for over a decade and have yet to have one complain about gaining too much muscle.

While it is true that some people can put on muscle much easier than others (everyone's body is unique), women simply do not have enough testosterone to bulk up with the amount of weight training I will be recommending. I think this fear arises from having seen female bodybuilders on television or in magazines.

These women put in a lot more time at the gym than you will be asked to. They lift extremely heavy weights frequently and eat a strictly regimented diet. Often the professional bodybuilders are supplementing all of this by using chemicals supplements, (some legal and some not) to offset the fact that their bodies do not naturally produce enough testosterone to build that much muscle. With just a little experience with lifting weights you will understand just how difficult it can be to add muscle mass.

Lifting Weights Will Increase Your Metabolism

You may be saying to yourself, "I'm not trying to get muscular, I just want to get thinner and lose weight – why should I lift weights?" Lifting weights will help you get leaner, thinner, and lose weight. There are many benefits to weight lifting, but for the purposes of losing weight the biggest reason is that it can dramatically increase your metabolism! The best kept secret in weight loss is that the more muscle mass you have, the faster your metabolism will be.

Metabolism is the rate at which your body burns calories. So if your normal metabolic rate has your body burning 1,500 calories a day, if you can increase your metabolic rate by 10%, you will burn 1,650 calories a day. As you can imagine, this can be extremely helpful when you are trying to lose weight. In a perfect world, we would all be genetically gifted and have turbocharged metabolisms, making it easy to maintain a healthy weight. The next best thing in the real world is to gain lean muscle mass to help you crank up your metabolism.

You can also boost your metabolism with some dietary modifications, which we will discuss in detail in the nutrition chapter.

Losing Pounds Versus Losing Inches

Remember, muscle weighs more than fat. As we discussed in the goal setting chapter, it is common for someone to start an exercise program, do great and lose dress sizes, but their weight to not drop significantly. This will often happen because the person is gaining lean muscle at the same time they are losing fat.

So before you panic or get frustrated if your weight does not drop as rapidly as you had hoped, first evaluate how your clothes are fitting. If your clothes have suddenly gotten a lot looser, then fantastic, you are on your way. The most important aspects on your weight loss journey are your size and measurements changing! After all, isn't that what you are after – to improve the way you look and how your clothes fit?

Weight Training – Overview

Later in this chapter there are a list of specific weight training exercises that I recommend, along with photos and descriptions that show the proper form for each exercise. We will also discuss some detailed weight training advice for beginner, intermediate, and advanced weight trainers, including number of sets, number of repetitions, amount of weight, and how often you should weight train.

Importance of Proper Form

Before we get into those specific details, let's discuss some weightlifting basics that apply to everyone. First and foremost, I cannot emphasize enough how important correct form is when you are weightlifting. At best, failure to use proper form can keep you from getting the full benefit from the exercise. At worst, improper form can result in injury and totally sidetrack you from your weight loss efforts. I say this not to scare you, but to emphasize the importance of good form.

As long as you review the photos later in this chapter and follow the instructions given, your form should be fine and you won't have any problems. If you can afford it, you can also hire a personal trainer for a few sessions to walk you through the different exercises. If you want a lower cost option, try out my free trial membership offer at www.GetRealZone.com and check out the online videos so you can get an even better view of proper form for each exercise.

I also recommend that you check out the anatomy chart in the appendix to learn the locations of the different muscles. You don't need to memorize every muscle in the body, just become familiar with the major muscles in the arms, legs, and torso. A basic understanding of the major muscle groups will help you to more effectively work out your body. When you know what body part you are working with a particular exercise, you will find it easier to isolate those muscles and use proper form. If you just go through the motions without knowing precisely what you are targeting, your efforts will be less effective. The mind-body connection will help you get better results!

Drink Plenty of Water During Your Workouts

Another key issue when lifting weights is to drink water frequently. Every gym has water fountains so take a quick water break at least every ten minutes or so. If you are exercising at home make sure you keep a water bottle nearby. Even though you may not be sweating as much as you will during cardio, you still need to stay hydrated while lifting weights.

Soreness

Soreness is a very big issue for many beginners, most of whom will feel at least slightly sore initially. Depending on how out of shape you are you may feel extremely sore at first, as it varies a lot among individuals. The key point to remember is that it is okay to be sore. Do not get discouraged. Your body is just getting used to the new workload it is being given. If you just give it a couple of weeks to adapt, you will really feel it coming together as your body gets used to the lifting.

The most common reaction to soreness is to try to avoid movement because it is somewhat uncomfortable. But actually the best thing you can do is to get moving! For example, if you are sore when you begin doing your cardio, you will feel much better and looser at the end of your workout.

The movement helps burn off the lactic acid in your muscles which causes the soreness. Have you ever gotten up in the morning and felt only slightly sore and then been extremely sore after sitting at your desk all day? The reason for that is the lactic acid has built up and there has been no movement to help you rid your muscles of it. So the lesson is to get moving and the soreness will disappear!

Weight Training Skill Levels

Just like cardiovascular exercise, everyone who lifts weights fits into one of three categories, beginner, intermediate, and advanced. For our purposes, a weight training beginner is someone who has never lifted weights or who has not done any weight training in the past six months or more. An intermediate is someone who does weight training either occasionally (maybe twice a week) or inconsistently, but does not let more than a week or so pass between weight training sessions. Finally, the advanced weight trainer is one who consistently lifts weights at least three times per week. An advanced person is not necessarily an athlete, but is simply more consistent about weight training than the other groups. Depending on what category you fall under, follow the detailed instructions given below on how to structure your workouts.

Preparation and Planning Your Workouts

First, let's start with some definitions for the true beginner. In weightlifting there are exercises, sets, and repetitions. An exercise is the actual body movement that you do. For example, you do lat pull downs to work your latissimus dorsi (the large back muscles). A repetition, or "rep," is a single motion of an exercise. A single lat pull down would be one repetition or rep. A "set" is a group of reps done without stopping. So if you did two sets of lat pull downs with ten reps each, that means you did ten lat pull downs, you stopped and rested for 30 to 90 seconds, then you did another set of ten lat pull downs. This will be important to understand when you begin to design your workouts later in this chapter.

Below is a list of some of the most useful and common exercises so that you can create your own full body workout. It is important to exercise all the major muscles to help build overall strength and prevent muscle imbalances. For each muscle group, there are 2 - 4 exercises shown using dumbbells as well as machines and equipment likely to be found at most gyms. A sufficient assortment of exercises is given that will allow you to create workouts that can be done either at the gym or at home.

Focus on Form While Using Dumbbells

One quick note about working out with dumbbells – maintaining proper form when exercising with dumbbells is a little more difficult compared to using most exercise machines. This is because you do not have a machine that is placing you in the proper position and forcing you to use proper form. Instead of the machine holding you in place, you must use other stabilizing muscles (not those directly involved in the exercise) to maintain your form.

How Much Time In Between Sets?

When you begin to do your workouts it is important that you give yourself a sufficient break between sets, but not too much. Between each set you should rest for 30 to 90 seconds. The heavier the weight you are working out with, the longer the rest period. I recommend actually looking at your watch to time yourself between sets initially, until you get a feel for how much time you should rest in between sets.

How Much Weight Should You Use?

Here is a general rule for determining how much weight you should use for a given exercise. The proper weight will be heavy enough that, using proper form and the full range of motion, you cannot do more than 15 repetitions, but not so heavy that you are unable to do at least ten reps. In short, you should be able to do 10-15 repetitions and by the last 2-3 reps you should have some difficulty and really be feeling the burn. If toward the end of the set you find that you are unable to maintain proper form, then you need to lower the weight. On the other hand, if you don't feel difficulty by rep 15, you need to increase the weight.

There are some details of weight training that are unique for each of the three levels. Below, based on your level, is an outline explaining the number of sets and repetitions to do, how frequently you should do weight training, and how to structure and plan the actual workout.

Guidelines for Weight Lifting Beginners

Number of Sets:

For beginners, you should do one set of each exercise for the first week. Then the following week, once your body has been introduced to lifting, increase it to two sets per exercise.

Number of Repetitions:

12 to 15 repetitions – It is better to perform more reps at first. Using lighter weights will help ensure you have good form.

Frequency and Scheduling of Weight Training Sessions:

Beginners should lift weights at least two times per week, preferably three. Anything less than two is simply not enough to get sufficient results. However, weight training workouts should not be performed on consecutive days to allow the muscles at least 24 hours of recovery time. For example, if you worked out on a Monday you should not work out again until Wednesday.

How to Plan and Select the Exercises:

Planning the workouts is extremely simple for beginners – for each workout you should do one exercise for each muscle group. So just pick one of exercises listed below for each category and, voila, there is your workout plan. A sample beginner workout is shown below.

Sample Beginner's Workout

Muscle	Exercise	# Sets	# of Reps
Glutes	Lunges	1	8-10 per leg
Chest	Push Ups	1	8-10*
Quadriceps	Leg Extensions	1	12
Back	Lat Pull Down	1	12
Hamstrings	Leg Curl (machine)	1	12
Shoulder	Shoulder Press	1	12
Abdominals	Crunches (on the floor)	1	15
Triceps	Tricep Pushdowns	1	12
Calves	Calf Raises – Standing	1	12-15

*Knees down for women and conventional for men; fewer reps are listed for beginners because of the difficulty level.

Guidelines for Weight Lifting Intermediates

Number of Sets:

For intermediates, you should do at least two

sets of each exercise, and then increase to three sets as your conditioning improves.

Number of Repetitions:

10-12 repetitions – Since you are acclimated to the exercises and the proper form, you can use slightly heavier weight and do fewer repetitions.

Frequency and Scheduling of Weight Training Sessions:

You should lift weights three times per week. However, your workouts should be planned to allow at least 24-48 hours between workouts engaging the same muscle groups, to give those specific muscles sufficient recovery time. That will make your workout planning somewhat more complicated than for the beginners, but not to worry. This is easily handled by doing different body parts on different days. For example, you could do upper body on Monday, lower body on Wednesday, and upper and lower body combination on Friday. The key is to schedule your workouts in a way that has you working your rested muscles while allowing your sore muscles time to recover.

How to Plan and Select the Exercises:

After you determine what body parts you will be exercising on what days, the planning becomes fairly simple. Just select one or two exercises for the appropriate body parts for that day and there is your workout plan. As an intermediate you should do at least two sets of each exercise. When this is not challenging enough, increase the number of sets per exercise to three. The sample week's worth of workout plans below will give you a good idea of how this should be structured.

Sample Workouts for Intermediates

Workout #1

Muscle	Exercise	# Sets	# of Reps
Back	Lat Pulldown	2	12
Chest	Flyes	2	10
Shoulder	Shoulder Press	2	12
Back	Seated Row	2	12
Chest	Incline Chest Press	2	12
Shoulder	Lateral Shoulder Raises	2	10
Triceps	Tricep Extensions	2	12
Biceps	Hammer Curls	2	12
Abdominals	Crunches on the Floor	2	15

Workout #2

Muscle	Exercise	# Sets	# of Reps
Abdominals	Crunches on Stability Ball	2	12
Glutes	Squats	2	10

Muscle	Exercise	# Sets	# of Reps
Hamstrings	Straight Leg Deadlifts	2	10
Quadriceps	Leg Press	2	12
Abdominals	Crunches Using Medicine Ball	2	10 per side
Glutes	Lunges	2	10 per leg
Hamstrings	Leg Curl – Stability Ball	2	10
Quadriceps	Leg Extensions	2	12
Calves	Standing Calf Raises	2	12-15

Guidelines for Advanced Weight Lifters

Number of Sets:

For advanced weight trainers, you should do at least three sets of each exercise and then increase to four sets as your conditioning improves.

Number of Repetitions:

8-10 repetitions – As you become stronger and are comfortable with the exercises it is safe and beneficial to push yourself more by lifting heavier and reducing the number of reps.

Frequency and Scheduling of Weight Training Sessions:

You should lift weights three or four times per week. I should note that it is counterproductive to lift weights more than four or five times a week, as it is possible to over train and not give your body sufficient time to recover.

As with intermediates, your workouts need to be at least 24 to 48 hours apart for each muscle that is worked, to allow those specific muscles sufficient recovery time. Since you will be doing more frequent workouts, this will require a bit more planning, but it is easily manageable. For example, you could do back and biceps on Monday, legs on Tuesday, chest, shoulders and triceps on Thursday, and some combination on Saturday.

How to Plan and Select the Exercises:

As with intermediate workouts, when you decide what body parts to work on what days the planning becomes fairly simple. Just select two to four exercises for the appropriate body parts for that day and your workout plan is done. As an advanced weight trainer you should do at least three sets of each exercise. When this is not challenging enough, either increase the number of sets per exercise to four or increase the amount of weight. The sample week's worth of workout plans below will give you a good idea of how this should be structured.

Sample Workouts for Advanced

Workout #1

Muscle	Exercise	# Sets	# of Reps
Back	Pull Ups*	3	8-10
Abdominals	Sit Ups on Decline Bench**	3	15
Back	Dumbbell Rows	3	10
Biceps	Hammer Curls	3	10
Abdominals	Crunches on the Floor**	3	20
Back	Lat Pulldowns	3	10
Biceps	Bicep Curl Machine	3	10

*Can be assisted by a spotter or using the assistance machine

**Abdominals can be done 4-5 times a week and reps can increase as strength increases

Workout #2

Muscle	Exercise	# Sets	# of Reps
Glutes	Squats	3	10
Hamstrings	Dead Lifts	3	10
Quadriceps	Leg Press	3	10
Calves	Calf Raises – Standing	3	10-15
Glutes	Lunges	3	10
Hamstrings	Leg Curl Machine	3	10
Quadriceps	Leg Extension	3	10
Calves	Calf Raises – Seated	3	10-15

Workout #3

Muscle	Exercise	# Sets	# of Reps
Chest	Push Ups – Conventional	3	10
Shoulders	Shoulder Press	3	10
Abdominals	Crunches- Obliques – On Stability Ball	3	10-15 per side
Chest	Bench Press	3	10
Triceps	Dips*	3	10
Shoulders	Anterior Shoulder Raises	3	10 per side
Shoulders	Reverse Flyes	3	10
Triceps	Tricep Extensions	3	10

*Can be assisted by a spotter or using the assistance machine

As you continue to follow the workout regimen you can increase the intensity by either lifting heavier weight or by doing more exercises per muscle group.

Now that you know how to plan your workouts, let's learn exactly how to do the specific exercises. On the next page is a list of the major muscle groups you will work out, along with several exercises to choose from for each muscle.

List of Exercises

Muscle Group	Exercises
Deltoids (Shoulder)	1. Shoulder Press 2. Lateral Shoulder Raise (bent arm) 3. Lateral Shoulder Raise (straight arm) 4. Anterior Shoulder Raise 5. Reverse Flyes
Latissimus Dorsi (Back)	1. Seated Row 2. Lat Pull Down 3. Pull Ups (outside grip) 4. Pull Ups (inside grip) 5. Dumbbell Row
Pectoralis (Chest)	1. Push Ups (knees down) 2. Push Ups (conventional) 3. Incline Chest Press 4. Bench Press 5. Flyes
Biceps	1. Bicep Curls 2. Hammer Curls
Triceps	1. Tricep Pushdowns 2. Tricep Extensions 3. Dips

Muscle Group	Exercises
Quadriceps (front of thigh)	1. Leg Extension 2. Leg Press
Gluteus (butt - also for the quadriceps)	1. Lunges 2. Squats
Hamstrings (back of thigh)	1. Leg Curl (machine) 2. Straight Leg Dead Lifts (dumbbells) 3. Leg Curl (using stability ball)
Calves (back of lower leg)	1. Calf Raises – Standing 2. Calf Raises – Seated
Abdominals	1. Crunches (on the floor) 2. Crunches (on the stability ball) 3. Crunches – Obliques (on stability ball) 4. Crunches – Oblique (using a medicine ball) 5. Sit ups (on a decline bench)

This list of exercises is just a few of the many possible exercises that can be performed for each body part. So if you are familiar with other exercises feel free to perform them. Because of the size limitations of this book it is impossible to give more than a few exercises for each, but check out www.GetRealZone.com for a free trial membership that will provide you with specific instructions on how to do many more exercises, many sample workouts, ideas for how to keep your workouts fresh and fun, and even video demonstrations of the exercises.

Deltoids (Shoulders) Exercise #1 –

Shoulder Press Using Dumbbells

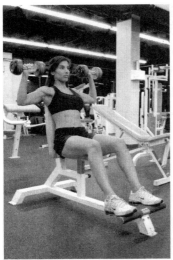 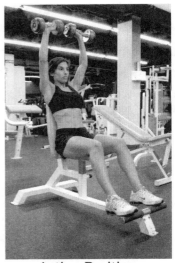

Start/End Position   Action Position

Description:

Hold weights above shoulders at ear level with palms facing forward.

Raise dumbbells up and inward above your head and then slowly lower weights to starting position.

Tips:

*Do not lock elbows at the top range of the motion.

*Do not sway weights back and forth.

*Keep back pressed firmly against bench throughout range of motion.

Deltoids (Shoulders) Exercise #2 –

Lateral Shoulder Raise With Bent Arm Using Dumbbells

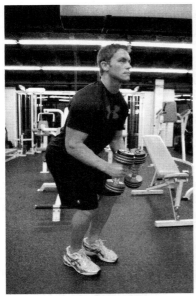 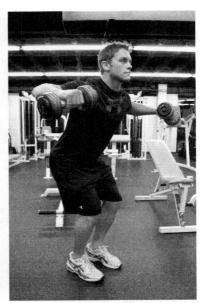

Start/End Position   Action Position

Description:

Stand with feet shoulder width apart, knees bent. Hold weights in front of you with elbows bent and palms facing inward. Lean forward, keeping your back straight and stomach in tight.

Raise the weights to your sides, keeping elbows bent until elbows are even with shoulders. Then lower dumbbells to start position.

Tip:

*At the top of the range shoulders, elbows, and hands should be in alignment. Elbows should not drop below your hands.

Deltoids (Shoulders) Exercise #3 –

Lateral Shoulder Raise with Straight Arm Using Dumbbells

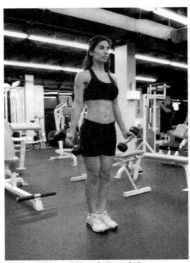
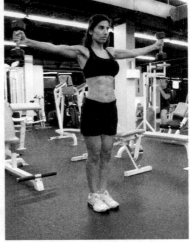

Start/End Position   Action Position

Description:

Stand upright with arms straight and hands directly to your sides with palms facing out.

Raise arms to shoulder level keeping your elbows locked and then lower the weights back down to start position.

Tip:

*Do not lean forward or backward while raising the dumbbells.

Deltoids (Shoulders) Exercise #4 –

Anterior Shoulder Raise Using Cable Machine

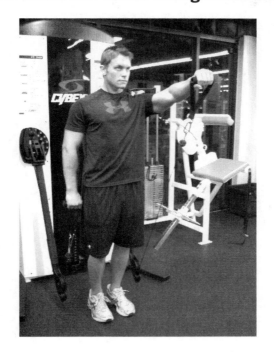

Description:

Start – stand upright with feet slightly apart and stomach tight. Hold cable (or dumbbells) in hand with palms facing down.

Action – raise arm to shoulder level, keeping arm straight and back straight. This exercise can be performed with one arm at a time or together.

Tip:

*Be careful not to sway backward when raising the weights, especially when lifting both sides together.

Deltoids (Shoulders) Exercise #5 –

Reverse Flyes Using Dumbbells

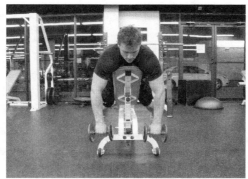

Start/End Position

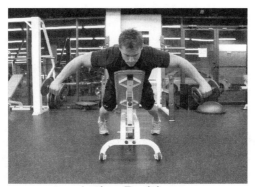

Action Position

Description:

Place chest on a bench (in the incline position) with both feet on the floor. Let arms hang straight down with palms facing you.

Raise the dumbbells to your sides (while keeping elbows bent) until your elbows reach shoulder level. Then slowly lower weights back to the start position.

Tip:

*Do not lift chest off bench when raising dumbbells.

Latissimus Dorsi (Back) – Exercise #1

Seated Row Using Cable Machine

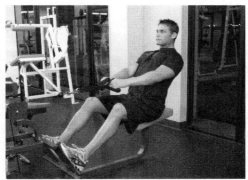

Start/End Position

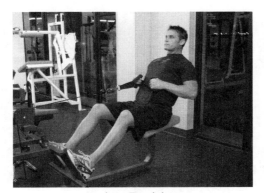

Action Position

Description:

Hold the cable with palms facing in, lean back (without arching back) and stomach tight.

Pull cable in towards chest while keeping elbows close in and not flared out.

Tip:

*Do not sway back as you pull the weights toward you.

Latissimus Dorsi (Back) – Exercise #2

Lat Pulldown Machine

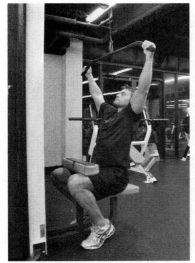 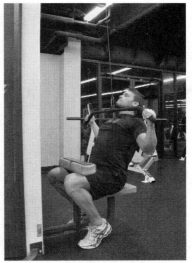

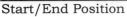

Start/End Position   Action Position

Description:

While seated on machine place your thighs securely under the knee pads. Hold the bar with a wide grip.

Pull the bar down to the top of your chest. Keep your elbows below the bar.

Tip:

*Do not lean further back as you pull the bar down.

Latissimus Dorsi (Back) – Exercise #3

Pull Ups (Outside Grip)

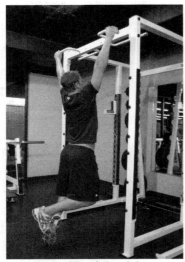 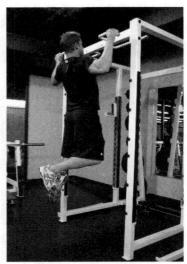

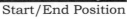

Start/End Position   Action Position

Description:

Grasp the handles and keep stomach tight. Pull chin up to the bar while keeping your elbows out to the sides.

Tips:

*Do not swing your body back in order to raise yourself up.

*If you are unable to perform the pull up you can use the assisted pull up machine or have someone assist you by spotting you from your shins or waist.

Latissimus Dorsi (Back) – Exercise #4

Pull Ups (Inside Grip)

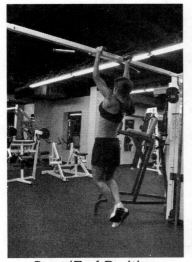

Start/End Position   Action Position

Description:

Grasp the inside handles with palms facing inward. Lift chin up to the bar and lower back to starting position without locking elbows.

Tip:

*Do not swing body to raise yourself up.

Latissimus Dorsi (Back) – Exercise #5

Dumbbell Row

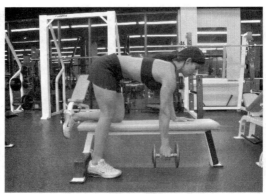

Start/End Position

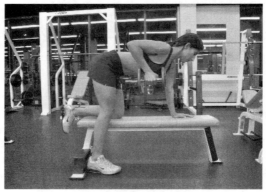

Action Position

Description:

Kneel on the bench with your left knee and support your upper body by placing your left hand on the bench (directly under left shoulder). Be sure that your back is straight and parallel to the floor and hold your abs in tight. Hold a dumbbell in your right hand and let your arm hang down and fully extend.

Pull the dumbbell up to your chest, keeping your elbow in close. Pause at the top and then lower weight back to the start position. After completing the set, repeat on the other side.

Tip:

*Do not move your back up and down as you raise and lower the weight. Back should remain straight.

Pectoralis (Chest) – Exercise #1

Push Ups (Knees Down)

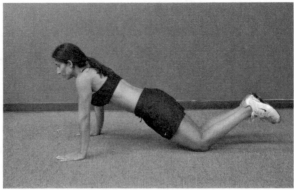

Start/End Position

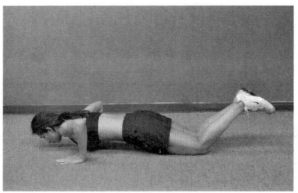

Action Position

Description:

Kneel down on the floor and place hands directly below your shoulders. Hold the stomach in tight and keep your back straight without dropping or raising the hips.

Lower your chest to the floor directly between your hands. As you lower yourself, let your elbows fall out to the sides. Then raise yourself back to the starting position.

Tip:

Do not hold elbows close in when lowering your body – this puts undue stress on the shoulders.

Pectoralis (Chest) – Exercise #2

Push Ups (Conventional)

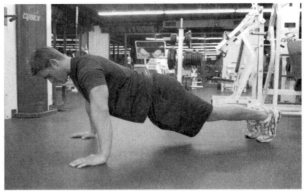

Start/End Position

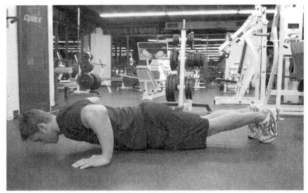

Action Position

Description:

Place your hands and feet on the floor, with your hands below the shoulders. Hold your stomach in tight and keep your back straight. Do not drop or raise your hips.

Lower your chest to the floor between your hands. Then raise yourself back up to the start position.

*The conventional push up is more difficult than the knees down push up.

Pectoralis (Chest) – Exercise #3

Incline Chest Press

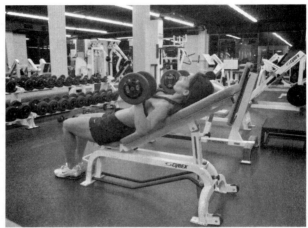

Start/End Position

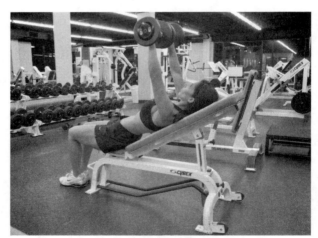

Action Position

Description:

Lie on a bench in the incline position. Hold the dumbbells at chest level with palms facing forward.

Raise the weights over your chest, bringing them up and together. Then slowly lower the dumbbells to the sides of your chest (but not below the chest level).

Tip:

*Do not arch your back when lifting the weights up.

Pectoralis (Chest) – Exercise #4

Bench Press

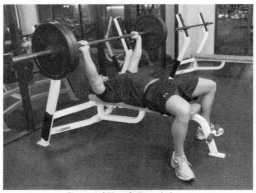

Start/End Position

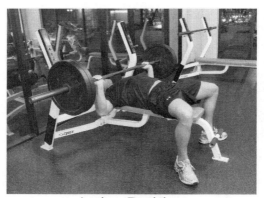

Action Position

Description:

Lie down on a flat bench. Hold the bar placing your hands directly above your shoulders, or slightly wider.

Lift the bar from the rack and lower the bar down to your chest. Then raise the bar back up without locking your elbows.

Tips:

*Do not arch your back when raising the weight back up. Back should remain flat on the bench.

*Caution: the bench press should never be done without a spotter!

Pectoralis (Chest) – Exercise #5

Flyes

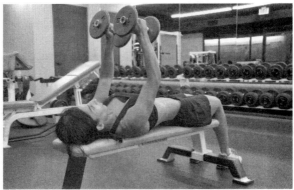

Start/End Position

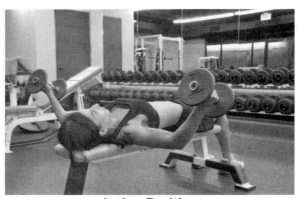

Action Position

Description:

Lie down on a flat bench. Hold the dumbbells above your chest with palms facing in. Keep a slight bend in your arms and do not lock your elbows.

Lower the dumbbells to your sides, maintaining the bend in your elbows. Lower the weights until your upper arm is parallel to the floor and elbows are even with shoulders.

Tip:

*Do not arch your back as you raise and lower the weight.

Biceps – Exercise #1

Bicep Curl Machine

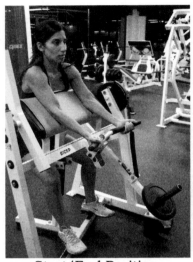 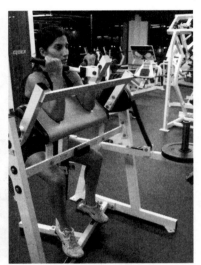

Start/End Position   Action Position

Description:

Sit on seat and place upper arms on pad making sure your elbow is even with the fulcrum point. Grab the handles and keep shoulders square and chest up.

Raise the handles toward your shoulders, squeeze the bicep muscle, and then lower the bar back to the starting position without locking your elbows.

Tip:

*Do not move your chest off the pad as you lift the weight towards you.

Biceps – Exercise #2

Hammer Curls

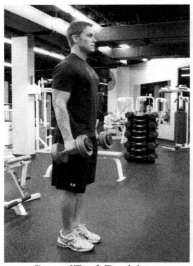 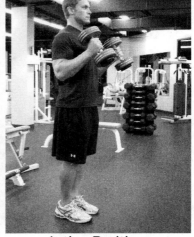

Start/End Position   Action Position

Description:

Stand straight with your stomach tight. Grasp a dumbbell in each hand and hold the weights to your side with your palms facing inward.

Curl both arms, lifting the dumbbells to your shoulders. Make sure to keep your elbows locked to your sides while lifting the weight. Then lower the dumbbell to the starting position.

Tip:

*Do not lean torso back as you lift the weight. Keep back straight at all times.

Triceps – Exercise #1

Tricep Pushdowns Using Cable

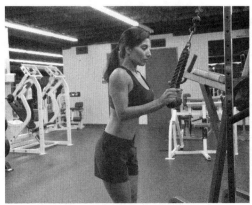

Start/End Position

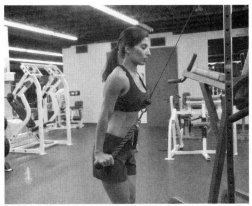

Action Position

Description:

Position the cable high and grab the rope at two ends. Lean torso slightly forward and keep elbows locked to your sides at all times. Forearms should be at 90° or slightly above.

Pull the cable rope down to the thighs or hips (for increased difficulty). Make sure to squeeze the tricep muscle at the bottom of the range of motion.

Tips:

*Do not move elbows while raising or lowering the weight and be sure to keep your torso stable with abs tight.

*Do not bend wrists forward or back while raising or lowering the weight.

Triceps – Exercise #2

Triceps Extension Using Dumbbells

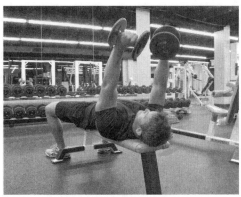

Start/End Position

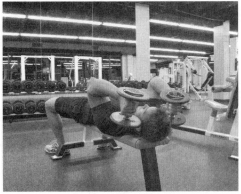

Action Position

Description:

Lie down on a flat bench. Hold a dumbbell in each hand, directly over your shoulder.

With your palms facing inward, lower the dumbbell to the sides of your head. Then raise them back to the starting position.

Tip:

*Keep elbows in place and do not let them flare out or move forward while raising the weight back up.

Triceps – Exercise #3

Dips

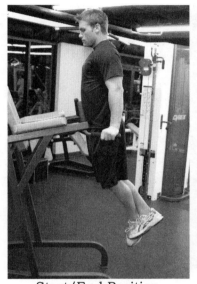 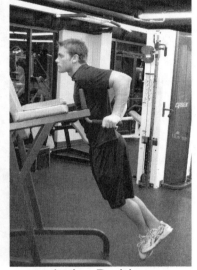

Start/End Position   Action Position

Description:

Grab handles and extend arms fully. Place your hands directly below the shoulders.

Lower your body while leaning forward slightly. Do not drop shoulders below elbow level (this puts unnecessary stress on shoulders). Extend arms fully and squeeze the tricep muscle at the top of the range of motion.

Tip:

*Do not sway body back and forth while raising and lowering yourself.

Quadriceps (Front of Thigh) – Exercise #1

Leg Extension Machine

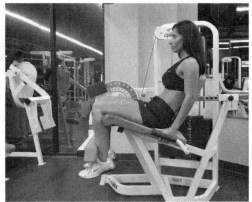

Start/End Position

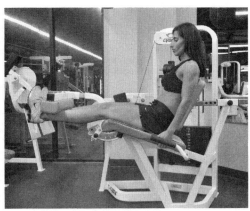

Action Position

Description:

Sit on the machine and place your legs under the padded bar. Feet should be positioned directly under the knees.

Raise the bar up until legs are fully extended. Hold onto the seat or handles so your hips do not raise upward. Then lower the weight all the way down to the start position.

Tip:

*Do not perform the exercise fast. Be sure to lower and raise the weight in a slow and controlled fashion.

Quadriceps (Front of Thigh) – Exercise #2

Leg Press

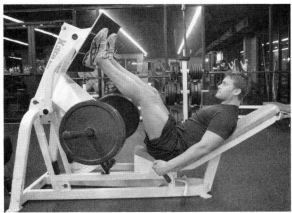

Start/End Position

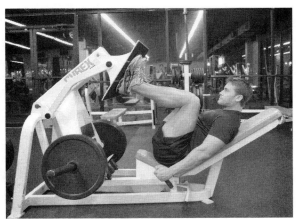

Action Position

Description:

Seat yourself on the machine. Place your feet on the platform about hip width apart.

Lower the weight to where your thighs touch your stomach. Then extend legs up again to start position without locking your knees.

Tip:

*Do not lock your knees at the top of the range of motion.

Gluteus (Butt) – Exercise #1

Lunges

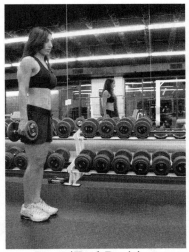 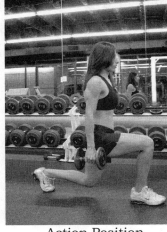

Start/End Position   Action Position

Description:

Stand straight with your feet together and a dumbbell in each hand (for beginners, perform the exercise without dumbbells).

Lunge forward with your right leg. Front and back leg should each be at 90°. Be sure that your right knee does not extend past your right toes. Then push off of your right foot and place leg back to start position. Alternate lunges with right and left leg.

Tips:

*Do not drop your chest and shoulders when stepping forward.

*Keep your back straight at all times.

Gluteus (Butt) – Exercise #2 –

Squats with a Barbell

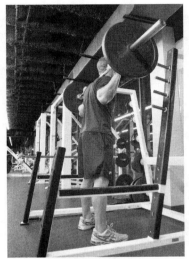
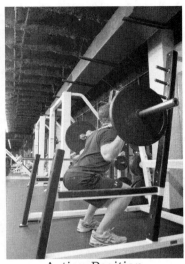

Start/End Position   Action Position

Description:

Stand straight with your feet shoulder width apart. Place barbell on back of the shoulders (not the neck) and hold the bar with a wide grip outside your shoulders.

Lower yourself by bending your knees to the point where your thighs are parallel to the floor. Be sure to keep your chest up and back as straight as possible.

Tip:

*Do not lean forward by dropping your chest when you bend down (this strains the back).

Hamstring (Back of Thigh) – Exercise #1

Leg Curl Machine

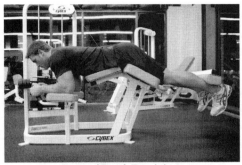

Start/End Position

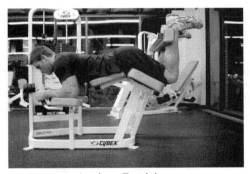

Action Position

Description:

Lie down on machine, placing the padded bar over your ankles.

Curl your legs up so the pad almost touches or does touch the back of your thighs.

Tip:

*Do not lift your glutes up as your pull the weight up.

Hamstring (Back of Thigh) – Exercise #2

Straight Leg Dead Lifts w/Dumbbells

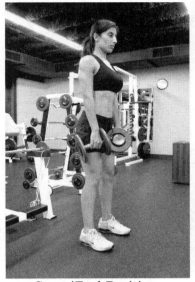 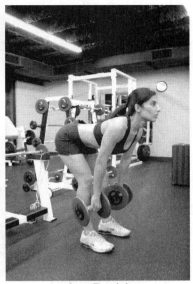

Start/End Position   Action Position

Description:

Stand with your back straight, stomach in, shoulders back and chest out throughout the range of motion. Keep your feet shoulder width apart with a dumbbell in each hand.

Bend forward at the hips and slowly lower the weights to your shins. Then slowly rise back up to the starting position. Be sure to keep the weights close to you and not far out in front of you.

Tip:

*Do not arch your back or bend your knees as you bend forward – only flexion is at the hip joint.

Hamstring (Back of Thigh) – Exercise #3

Leg Curl Using Stability Ball

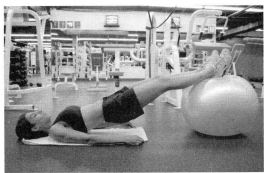

Start/End Position

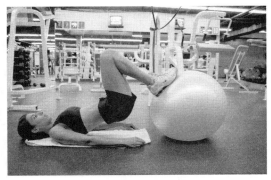

Action Position

Description:

Lie on the floor and place your calves on a stability ball. Then raise your hips up (the less leg/calf touching the ball the higher the level of difficulty and the more leg/calf touching the ball the lower the level of difficulty).

While keeping your hips up, roll the ball in towards your glutes and squeeze the glutes and hamstrings. Then extend your legs back out while keeping the hips up.

Tip:

*Do not lower your hips until you have completed the entire set.

Calves (Back of Lower Leg) – Exercise #1

Standing Calf Raise Machine

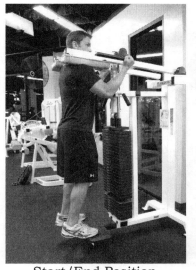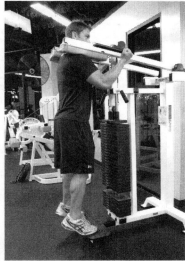

Start/End Position   Action Position

Description:

Stand straight with your shoulders under the pad and place the balls of your feet on the platform.

While keeping your knees locked, rise up and squeeze your calves. Then lower back down to the start position.

Tip:

*Do not lean forward when performing the exercise; keep your back straight.

Calves (Back of Lower Leg) – Exercise #2

Seated Calf Raise Machine

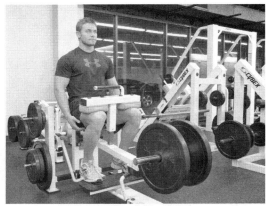

Start/End Position

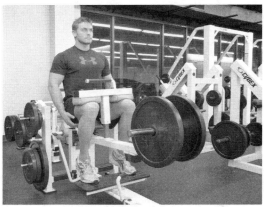

Action Position

Description:

Be seated on the machine with the pad on your lower thighs. Place the balls of your feet on the platform.

Raise the weight as high as you can and squeeze your calves and then lower back down.

Tip:

*Do not lean forward or back – keep your back straight.

Abdominals – Exercise #1

Crunches on the Floor

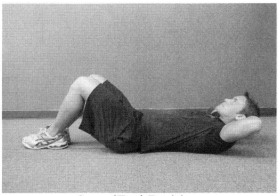

Start/End Position

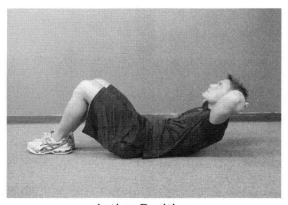

Action Position

Description:

Lie on the floor with your knees bent. Place your hands behind your head (without pulling on your head) and keep your elbows back.

Crunch up, pause, and squeeze your abdominals. Then lower yourself down without letting your shoulders touch the floor between repetitions.

Tips:

*This exercise has a small range of motion.

*Do not bend your neck when doing the crunches and keep your chin up at all times.

Abdominals – Exercise #2

Crunches on the Stability Ball

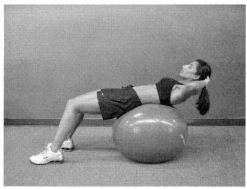

Start/End Position

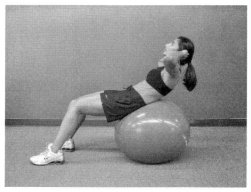

Action Position

Description:

Lie back on the ball with your shoulders, hips, and knees in a parallel line. Place your hands behind or on the side of your head (elbows back).

Crunch up and squeeze your abdominals. Be sure to keep your hips up and your chin up while crunching, then lower back down.

Tips:

*Do not sit up all the way at the top of the range of motion. Perform the exercise as pictured – this will keep the abdominals contracted the entire time.

Abdominals – Exercise #3

Crunches on the Stability Ball – Obliques

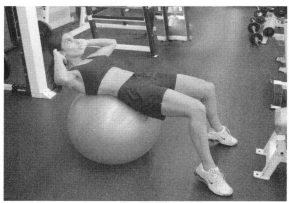

Start/End Position

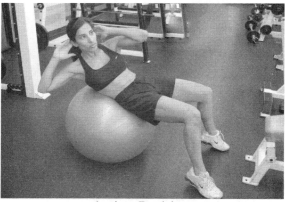

Action Position

Description:

This crunch targets your obliques (the sides of your abdomen). Use the same position as the previous crunch on the stability ball.

Crunch up raising your left elbow towards your right knee and squeeze your abs. Then lower back to the starting position and repeat on the same side.

Next do another set on the opposite side, lifting your right elbow towards your left knee.

Tip:

*Do not drop your hips while crunching up.

Abdominals – Exercise #4

Crunches Using a Medicine Ball (Obliques)

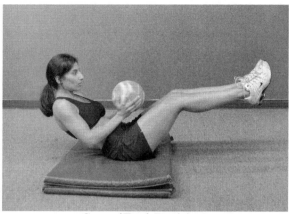

Start/End Position

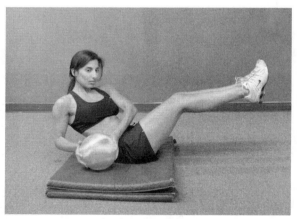

Action Position

Description:

Sit on the floor, tighten your abs, and with your back straight, lean back and raise feet off the floor (beginners can place feet on the floor with knees bent).

Twist using your obliques and tap the ball to the floor on each side (alternating sides). Keep arms bent and close in to your body.

Tip:

*Do not extend your arms out, thus making your arms work more and your obliques work less.

Abdominals – Exercise #5

Sit Ups on Decline Bench

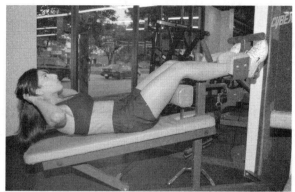

Start/End Position

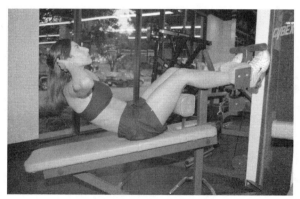

Action Position

Description:

Lie on the decline bench with your feet hooked in. Place your hands on the sides of your head and keep your chin up.

Crunch up half way, contract your abs and then lower slowly back down to the start position.

Tip:

*Do not go all the way up or come all the way back down onto the bench. Your abdominals should remain contracted until you have completed the entire set.

Chapter 7

Flexibility Training

Although flexibility is not directly associated with weight loss, it is an important part of a well balanced exercise regimen. Since you will be working out so hard (hint, hint...), you are likely to experience some soreness and stiffness from time to time. Stretching will help alleviate that discomfort.

The most beneficial time to stretch is immediately after exercising. This is because your muscles are already warmed up and therefore more pliable.

A common stretching mistake is to stretch in a bouncing fashion. This can result in an injury. The correct technique is to gently stretch to the point where you feel it, but it is not painful. More flexibility can be gained by holding the stretch for at least 15 seconds.

The following is an outline of some basic stretches for all the muscle groups. Be sure to follow the descriptions as well as the illustrations.

List of Stretches

Muscle Group	Stretch
Back	1. Cobra stretch 2. Cat Stretch 3. Side Twist
Quadriceps	1. Foot to Glute 2. Laying Foot to Glute
Hamstrings	1. Raised Straight Leg Hamstring Stretch
Gluteus	1. Standing Ankle on the Knee 2. Laying Ankle on the Knee
Calves	1. Raised Toes Calf Stretch (standard) 2. Raised Toes Calf Stretch (deeper)
Pectoralis (Chest)	1. Standing Chest Stretch
Triceps	1. Tricep Stretch 2. Tricep Side Stretch

Muscle Group	Stretch
Neck and Shoulder	1. Side Neck Stretch

Back Stretch #1 –

Cobra Stretch

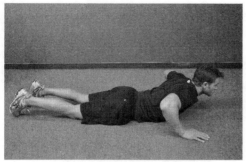

Start/End Position

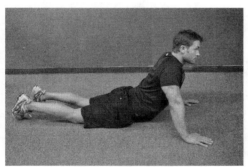

Action Position

Description:

Lie on the floor with your hands positioned just outside your chest.

Raise your chest up while keeping the pelvis in contact with the floor. You should feel the stretch in your lower back. Hold the stretch for

ten to fifteen seconds and repeat at least one to
two times.

Back Stretch #2 –

Cat Stretch

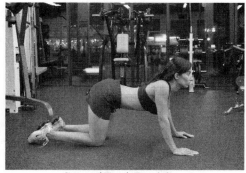

Start/End Position

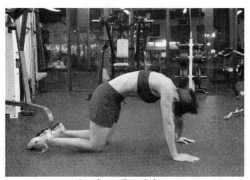

Action Position

Description:

Position yourself on the floor on all fours. Your knees should be directly under your hips and your hands should be below your shoulders.

Raise your back as high as you can, creating an arch while relaxing your neck and dropping your head down. Then lower your back down while raising your hips and lifting your head back up. Hold the stretch for ten to fifteen seconds and repeat at least one to two times.

Back Stretch #3 –

Side Twist

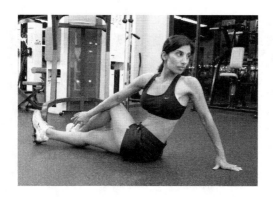

Description:

Be seated on the floor with your legs extended in front of you. Bend your left leg over your right leg and place your right elbow on the outside of your left knee and twist (looking behind you). Hold the stretch for ten to fifteen seconds and repeat at least one to two times for each side.

Quadricep Stretch #1 –

Foot to Glute

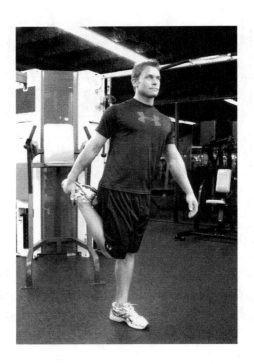

Description:

Stand upright. If you have trouble balancing you can stabilize yourself by holding something with your free hand.

Grasp your right foot with your right hand and pull your foot up to your glutes, while keeping your knees close together. You should feel the stretch in the front of your thigh. Hold the stretch for ten to fifteen seconds and repeat at least one to two times for each side.

Quadriceps Stretch #2 –

Laying Foot to Glute

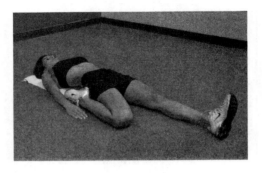

Description:

Lie on the floor and bend your right leg back until your foot touches your right glute. You should feel the stretch on the front of your thigh. Hold the stretch for ten to fifteen seconds and repeat at least one to two times for each side.

For a less intense stretch, do not lie flat but instead, rest your torso back on both elbows, thus elevating your torso (not shown).

*Caution: do not do this stretch if you have knee problems

Hamstring Stretch –

Raised Straight Leg Hamstring Stretch

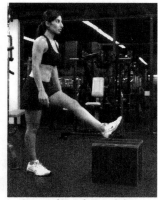

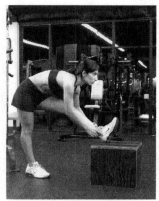

Start/End Position   Action Position

Description:

Stand straight and place your foot on a chair or bench with your toes pointing up and both knees locked. Slowly bend forward until you feel the stretch in the back of your thigh. Hold the stretch for ten to fifteen seconds and repeat at least one to two times for each side.

Gluteus Stretch #1 –

Standing Ankle on the Knee

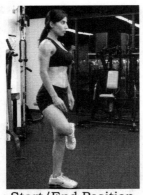
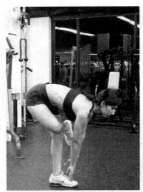

Start/End Position   Action Position

Description:

Stand straight and bend right leg over the left leg (above the knee). While keeping the stomach drawn in, bend forward without arching your back. Lean down as far as you are able (either to the shin, foot, or floor). Hold the stretch for ten to fifteen seconds and repeat at least one to two times for each side.

Gluteus Stretch #2 –

Laying Ankle on the Knee

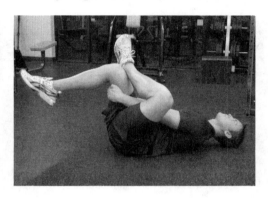

Description:

Lie down on the floor. Bend your right leg and cross your left leg over the right (above the knee). With both hands behind the right thigh, pull your right leg in towards you. Hold and repeat on opposite side. You should feel the stretch in your glutes. Hold the stretch for ten to fifteen seconds and repeat at least one to two times for each side.

Calf Stretch #1 –

Raised Toes Calf Stretch (Standard and Deep)

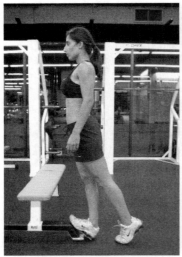 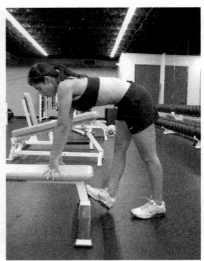

Standard Stretch   Deeper Stretch

Description:

Stand straight and place your foot against a ledge or wall, with your heel on the floor and your toes elevated. Shift your bodyweight forward, feeling the stretch in your calf. Hold the stretch for ten to fifteen seconds and repeat at least one to two times for each side.

For a deeper stretch lean forward further (as shown in photo above on the right).

Pectorals (Chest) Stretch –

Standing Chest Stretch

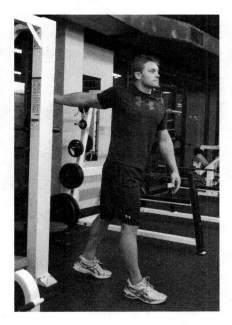

Description:

Standing straight, place right hand and arm back behind you with your right foot forward. Then slightly turn away – facing the left (keep extended arm straight). You should feel the stretch in your chest. Hold the stretch for ten to fifteen seconds and repeat at least one to two times for each side.

Triceps Stretches #1 –

Tricep Stretch

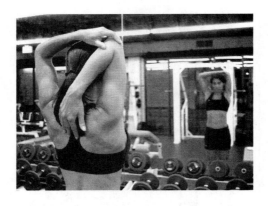

Description:

This stretch can be performed in a standing or seated position. Raise your right elbow so it points toward the ceiling and place your right hand between your shoulder blades. Then place your left hand on the right elbow and pull down. Hold the stretch for ten to fifteen seconds and repeat at least one to two times for each side.

Triceps Stretch #2 –

Tricep Side Stretch

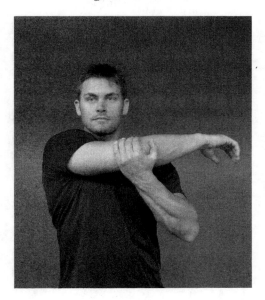

Description:

Extend your right arm across your body in front of you and pull your elbow in with your left hand. Hold the stretch for ten to fifteen seconds and repeat at least one to two times for each side.

Neck & Shoulder Stretch –

Side Neck Stretch

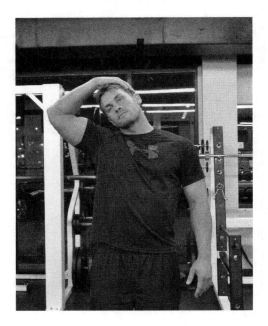

Description:

This stretch can be done standing or seated. Tilt your head to the right and place your right hand on your head and gently push down. You should feel the stretch along the left side of your neck. Hold the stretch for ten to fifteen seconds and repeat at least one to two times for each side.

Part Three –

Nutrition Simplified

Chapter 8

All About Nutrition –
Simplifying Carbohydrates,
Proteins, & Fats

There are two objectives for this section of the book. First, I want to provide some quick start tools that you can put to use right away that will help you start losing weight. Second, I want to teach you the basics of nutrition and healthy eating so that you can make informed eating decisions and become an "educated eater" who makes healthier diet decisions for the rest of your life.

When it comes to eating, people seem to have an endless number of questions. What should you eat? How much should you eat? How often should you eat? And many, many others.

This section will help to answer these questions and allow you to simplify your eating. Notice that I said "eating" and not dieting – the worst thing you can do is put yourself on an overly restrictive diet that requires you to completely eliminate certain food groups from your diet. Now I'm not about to tell you to eat anything you want, whenever you want it, but you do not need to give up anything completely.

Before we get to the quick start tools, let's first discuss the basics of nutrition so you not only know what you should do, but why you should do it.

Overview of Nutrition Basics

In order to fully comprehend how to eat a healthy diet that promotes weight loss we need to understand what makes up the food we eat. All foods fall primarily into one of three categories: carbohydrates, proteins, and fats.

Unlike some of the advice you may have gotten from the various fad diet literature, you need some of each of these categories in your daily diet. Where most overweight people have gone wrong is that they have failed to maintain a healthy balance between these three groups.

It has become too easy for all us hurried Americans to grab food on the go. Unfortunately, a lot of this food is highly processed and refined and is largely to blame for America's weight problem.

Carbohydrates

Contrary to popular belief, carbohydrates are not "bad" and they are not the enemy. Actually, our brains cannot function without carbohydrates. However, excess carbohydrates in your diet definitely are bad and this is one of the most common causes of weight gain.

A. *Different Kinds of Carbohydrates*

Let's discuss the different types of carbohydrates and how your body handles them. There are two types of carbohydrates: simple and complex. Simple carbohydrates are sugars and include sucrose (table sugar), fructose (found in fruit), and galactose (found in milk). Simple carbohydrates are digested quickly by our bodies. Complex carbohydrates are digested much more slowly, making them a much better choice for someone trying to lose weight.

When you eat carbs, your body converts them to glucose (sugar) to use as energy. The unused glucose is either stored in the liver as glycogen for energy or it is converted to fat and stored in the tissue. So if you eat too many carbs and you are not active enough to use them all up, your body will convert those unused carbs into fat – obviously, this is not what you want to have happen.

Another great reason to do weight training and other exercises that build muscle is that our muscle cells are much better at utilizing the sugar than our fat cells. In other words, a highly active person will burn off the excess sugar much more effectively than a sedentary person. The moral is that if you are overweight, then eating a diet high in carbohydrates will perpetuate your weight gain and, if you are sedentary, the situation is even worse.

B. Examples of Simple and Complex Carbohydrates

As described above, complex carbohydrates are generally a much better choice, so here are some examples of both simple and complex carbohydrates.

Simple Carbohydrates	Complex Carbohydrates
cakes	slow cooked oatmeal
cookies	potatoes and sweet potatoes
many cereals	whole wheat bread
chips	whole grain pasta
rice cakes	whole grain & high fiber cereal

Simple Carbohydrates	Complex Carbohydrates
most bread	brown and wild rice
jams	grains: quinoa, bulgur, millet, buckwheat
honey	cream of wheat, rice, rye
Chocolate/candy	lentils
soft drinks	tortillas – whole grain
fruits (but natural)	most vegetables

As you can probably tell from the list, the more processed the food is, the more likely it is to be a simple carbohydrate, and most "junk foods" are very high in simple carbohydrates.

Let me clarify a few of the items on this list. While I have listed vegetables as a complex carbohydrate, many of them do contain high amount of starch or sugar. Some of these high-starch vegetables are corn, carrots, butternut squash, peas, and potatoes. Please refer to the appendix for an extensive listing of the nutritional values for all of the most common vegetables.

You will note that many of the complex carbohydrates listed are "whole grain" products. Because of the somewhat confusing (and arguably misleading) packaging and marketing of many food products, many people have difficulty determining whether a food is truly whole grain. Here is what you should look for – on the product ingredients list it should include one of the following ingredients: whole wheat, whole oats, or some other whole grain. The key is to look for the word "whole." Preferably, this ingredient is listed first, meaning that it is the #1 ingredient in the product.

Many people are surprised that fruits are a simple carbohydrate. However, this does not mean you should avoid them, although while trying to lose weight you should limit yourself to two to three servings per day. Fruits are actually quite low in simple sugars and many fruits are very fibrous, which helps slow down the rate of their digestion.

There are some fruits that are better choices, however. For instance, fruits which have the highest sugar content, such as melons (cantaloupe and honeydew), mangoes, bananas, pineapples, and dried fruit, should be eaten in moderation. Please refer to the appendix for a complete list of nutritional values for most common fruits. Fruit juices should be avoided entirely. Though they may offer some nutrients, they have high amounts of sugar. The raw fruit makes a much better choice than its juice alone.

C. Advanced Issues with Carbohydrates

Although this a bit advanced, it is helpful to have a basic understanding of exactly how carbohydrates are broken down by your body. One measurement of how rapidly your body converts carbohydrates into glucose is the glycemic index. The glycemic index is a numerical value that tells you how fast the carbohydrates from a particular food affects your glucose level (also known as your blood sugar level). Simple carbohydrates that break down quickly have a high glycemic index, while complex carbohydrates that break down slowly have a low glycemic index.

Don't get overly concerned with the glycemic index. It rates individual foods and does not consider the effect the particular food has on blood sugar levels when consumed with other foods. For example, the effect of eating a potato alone as compared with eating a potato with some chicken results in a very different impact on blood sugar levels.

Another issue with how your body handles carbohydrates is how fast your glucose level rises. When your glucose level rises quickly, your body reacts by releasing insulin into your bloodstream to bring your glucose levels down to a normal level. This elevated insulin level in turn sends a message to your body to avoid burning any of its stored fat, directly resulting in weight gain.

Here is the typical chain of events for someone with a diet too high in carbs. A large quantity of simple carbs is consumed and digested very quickly, causing a spike in the glucose level. The body reacts by releasing insulin into the bloodstream to bring the blood sugar level back to normal. The elevated insulin level results in your body not burning the fat it is already storing. For many people this is a pattern that is repeated several times a day, resulting in significant weight gain.

Optimally, your glucose level should rise very slowly. You can make this process work much better by consuming complex carbohydrates in moderate amounts. Those carbohydrates will be digested much more slowly, thus avoiding both the spike in your glucose levels and the subsequent spike of insulin. This process is also helped by consuming high fiber foods, which are digested at a slower rate and keep you feeling full longer.

Proteins

Now that we've covered the basic chemistry behind carbohydrates, let's turn to protein.

A. Different Kinds of Protein

Proteins are comprised of amino acids. Some proteins are complete while others are incomplete. A complete protein is one that contains all the essential amino acids. These are amino acids your body requires but is incapable of producing on its own and, therefore, must obtain through the diet. An incomplete protein is simply one that does not contain all the essential amino acids.

Protein is found in foods such as eggs, nuts, meat, turkey, fish, tofu, lentils, and dairy products. Most meat proteins are complete proteins while most vegetable proteins are incomplete proteins. In terms of weight loss, the best forms of protein are the leaner varieties that have less fat.

B. Examples of Lean Protein and Fat Protein

To give you some dietary guidance, here are some examples of both lean proteins and higher-fat proteins. Please refer to the appendix for a detailed list of the nutritional content of some of the most common proteins.

Fat Protein	Lean Protein
80% ground beef	95% ground beef
ribeye steak	top sirloin/flank steak

Fat Protein	Lean Protein
corned beef	turkey breast
pork	chicken breast
lamb	most fish
duck	low fat cottage cheese
cheese (full fat)	low-fat cheese
tofu (heart healthy)	lentils
egg yolks	egg whites
sausage	veal
pepperoni	protein powder (whey, soy)
bacon	low fat yogurt
nuts	tofu (some varieties)

This list gives you an idea of how to make smart protein choices. This is not to say you can never have any of the "fat" proteins, but you should limit their consumption when you are trying to lose weight.

Here are a couple of notes to clarify some common areas of confusion about proteins.

When considering eating nuts you need to be aware of both the calories and fat, as you will need to cut back somewhere else in your diet in order to lose weight. With lentils, you need to be aware of the high content of complex carbohydrates. Thus, they should be consumed in smaller quantities than the other lean proteins.

Fat

Finally, let's discuss the different types of fat. Yes, even with fat, there are healthy and unhealthy varieties. The four types of fat are: saturated, monounsaturated, polyunsaturated, and hydrogenated (also known as trans fat).

A. Saturated Fats

Saturated fats are not good. They elevate the bad cholesterol (LDL) and triglyceride levels. Foods that are rich in saturated fats are fatty meat, skin on poultry, whole and 2% dairy products (milk, cheese, etc.), butter, coconut and palm oils.

B. Monounsaturated Fats

Monounsaturated fats are healthier for you. Monounsaturated fats help to lower your LDL cholesterol level (commonly referred to as the "bad" cholesterol). Monounsaturated fats also help to raise your HDL cholesterol level (HDL is the "good" cholesterol).

Monounsaturated fat can be found in: olive oil, canola oil, peanut oil, olives, avocados, and peanut butter (also other nut butters).

C. *Polyunsaturated Fats*

Polyunsaturated fat consists of two varieties, omega-3 and omega-6. Omega-3 is an essential fatty acid which has an anti-inflammatory effect on the body. This effect is of great importance because most diseases originate from some type of inflammatory response. The body is unable to make Omega-3 fatty acids on its own. Omega-3's can be found in fatty fish (salmon, sardines, mackerel, etc.) and in canola and soybean oils, flaxseeds/flaxseed oil, and walnuts.

Omega-6 fatty acids promote inflammation. They are found in: corn, soybean, sunflower and pumpkin seeds, and safflower oils. The omega-6 fats should be much more limited than the omega-3's.

D. Hydrogenated Fat (Trans Fat)

Finally the last fat to discuss is hydrogenated fat (also called trans fat). Hydrogenated fat is **not** a naturally occurring fat. It is a chemically engineered fat that becomes solid at room temperature. Examples of hydrogenated fats include margarine and vegetable shortening.

Often trans fat is added to packaged foods to prolong their shelf life. Some examples include crackers, cookies, and chips. Trans fats are even found in unlikely places such as seasonings, refrigerated or frozen breads, and many brands of peanut butter. The best way to avoid trans fats is to carefully read the "Nutrition Facts" label on food and look under the fat section for trans fats. If it says anything other than zero, you should avoid it.

E. How Much Fat Can You Consume

You should eat a single serving of the good fats (olives, avocados, nuts, and all natural nut butters) 3-4 times per week. In addition, you can have a single serving of low fat cheeses, flaxseeds/flaxseed and fish oils daily.

While trying to lose weight you really want to moderate your consumption of even the good fats. One of the primary reasons is the high level of calories contained in fat. Each gram of fat is equal to nine calories, while carbohydrates and protein each have only four calories per gram.

Now that you have a basic understanding of nutrition and how your body handles different kinds of food let's move on to specific eating plans and strategies.

Chapter 9

The Get Real Diet Plan –
How Much & How Often to Eat

A lot of people become confused and frustrated about exactly what they should eat when trying to lose weight. This is because most diets have very strict and complicated rules that are difficult to understand and consistently follow.

The Get Real Plan cuts through all of this and replaces it with simplicity. All you need to remember is that weight loss results from a net caloric deficit – if you consistently burn more calories than you consume you will lose weight. Understanding that simple concept and applying it to your daily life will lead to weight loss success, guaranteed.

If you are wondering how many calories you burn each day, it is important to understand that this number varies from person to person based on a number of different factors. Some of these factors are outside of your control, such as your gender (men generally burn more calories than women), your age (younger people generally burn more calories than older people), and your genes (a lucky few are born with relatively high metabolisms compared to the rest of us).

But other factors are completely within your control, such as how frequently you exercise and how much you exert yourself when you exercise. Those who exercise harder and longer will burn more calories than those who exercise sporadically and at a more modest exertion level.

So while there are a few factors that you can't alter, there is plenty within your control and certainly enough to reach your weight loss goal using the Get Real Plan!

The two most basic elements in weight loss are quite simply: 1) how many calories you burn and 2) how many calories you consume. In the beginning of this book you learned all about effective exercise and how it can dramatically increase the number of calories you burn. In the last chapter you learned the basics of nutrition and the different components of the food you eat. Now let's move on to the quantity and frequency of your food consumption.

Get Real Diet Plan

If you are worried that I am about to tell you to begin religiously counting calories or fat grams, fear not, the Get Real Diet Plan does not require it. Counting of calories, fat grams, carbohydrate grams, and fiber grams are not realistic strategies because life is simply too hectic to try to calculate these variables for every single thing that goes in your mouth.

Instead, all you need to do is follow the six Get Real Diet Plan Keys:

Get Real Diet Plan – Six Keys

1. Eat Consciously
2. Eat Five Small Meals a Day
3. Eat Three to Five Daily Servings of Vegetables
4. Eat a Hearty, Healthy Breakfast
5. Cheat in Moderation
6. Eat the Right Proportion of Protein, Carbs & Fat at Every Meal

Follow these six keys and you will be on the way to your target weight! Let's go into each of the keys in detail.

Get Real Diet Plan Key #1 –
Eat Consciously

The first step in learning how much to eat is learning to stop eating when we are full. This may sound like common sense, but consider how often you finish a meal and feel slightly or even very uncomfortable because you are too full. If you are like most people, this probably happens fairly often. Routinely overeating in this way is very common in our culture and a big factor that results in a calorie surplus and ultimately, weight gain.

Consider the difference between American and other cultures in this respect. Europeans, Mediterraneans, and Asians do not have some magical diet plan that keeps them thinner than Americans. But there are two big distinctions between their cultures and ours. The first is that these societies do not follow the "bigger is better" philosophy that is so pervasive in American diets. They do not "supersize" their meals, they simply eat until they are content.

The second distinction is that, unlike Americans, these cultures tend to slow down and enjoy their food. They do not rush their meals or eat on the go, the way that Americans so frequently do.

Here is why this matters. If you pay attention to your food and enjoy the tastes and textures, you will eat slower as a result and become conscious of when you are full. For example, if you eat a meal in front of the television you are likely to finish everything on your plate and not even realize it until you see that your plate is empty. The reason this happens is that your attention is diverted to what you are watching and not on what you are eating. You might even be full without realizing it because your brain has not had a chance to register it yet, since its focus was on the television program it was watching.

One of the ways you can really become conscious of what you are consuming is to keep a detailed daily food log. I recommend that you do this for at least a week when you begin the program. It will help keep you on track. See Appendix 4 for a sample food log. If you would like one you can print out and use to keep track of what you eat, visit GetRealZone.com/form2/.

The ultimate solution to eating without thinking is to sit down to eat your meals and actually pay attention to what is going in your mouth. Enjoy the texture and taste of the food and pay attention to when you begin to feel full. You may find yourself surprised at how quickly you get full and how much of a habit it has become to eat past the point of fullness. Do not eat meals in the car or at your desk or while doing some other task. Do this and you will really start to enjoy your food more without overeating.

Get Real Diet Plan Key #2 – Eat Five Smalls Meals a Day

Often people will try to lose weight by eating very infrequently, sometimes as little as once a day. They think the key to weight loss is will power and living with hunger. This is very counterproductive because though you have created a caloric deficit, you have also put your body into starvation mode so it will hold onto every calorie – not allowing for lasting weight loss.

The Get Real Plan requires you to eat five times a day – breakfast, morning snack, lunch, afternoon snack, and dinner. It may seem counterintuitive to eat this frequently, but it is one of the big keys to lasting success in weight loss.

When you eat three or fewer meals a day, you allow yourself to get very hungry. In turn, this tempts you to eat large portions of the wrong foods in one sitting to satisfy the hunger. When you eat a lot at once like this, your metabolism (the rate at which our bodies burn calories) slows down significantly. This is the opposite of what we want on our mission to create a net caloric deficit. We want our bodies burning calories at a rapid rate.

When you space out your meals and eat every three to four hours it allows your blood sugar levels to remain stable. As mentioned earlier, a spike in your blood sugar causes your insulin level to spike, which in turn promotes weight gain.

Thus, the lesson is that it is very important to eat small meals throughout the day. An added benefit is that you will feel more energized throughout the day, and you will avoid hitting those energy lulls and mood swings in the late afternoon. Finally, it will keep you from having unnecessary cravings for unhealthy foods because by the time you develop an appetite you will eat something small that will satisfy you until the next small meal. Eat on this schedule and you will find weight loss much simpler and easier.

Get Real Diet Plan Key #3 – Eat Three to Five Daily Servings of Vegetables

Not only is eating three to five daily servings of vegetables beneficial to overall good health, it will help you to reach your weight loss goal. Eating a variety of different colored vegetables will especially provide your body with more nutrients and prevent boredom of the same foods.

Please note that even though vegetables are primarily a carbohydrate (most have little protein or fat), under our plan they will not count as a carb (with a few exceptions noted below) and instead will be treated as a "freebie." You can have unlimited vegetables and I recommend that you have at least three servings a day. The reason why they are treated as a free food is that they are low in calories and, even though they are a carb, they contain very little sugar.

There is a tremendous selection of available vegetables so you really should expand your horizons and try some that are unfamiliar to you. You will likely stumble upon a few you like so much that they become staples of your diet.

In terms of nutritional content the best vegetables are fresh, followed closely by frozen, with canned coming in a distant third place. Among other problems with canned vegetables, the sodium content is extremely high. Preparing fresh vegetables is a lot simpler than most people realize, but if you really need convenience then go for frozen. They give you most of the benefit of fresh with less prep time.

The vegetables that do count as a carbohydrate are: corn, carrots, potatoes, squash, butternut squash, pumpkin, peas, and a few other uncommon vegetables. You should limit your consumption of these as they will count as a carbohydrate under the plan. Refer to Appendix 1 for the complete list.

Get Real Diet Plan Key #4 – Eat a Hearty, Healthy Breakfast

The old adage, "breakfast is the most important meal of the day," is not only true, it is a big key to achieving your weight loss goal. It is extremely common in our hurried culture to rush out the door without eating anything, justifying our behavior by saying that we are late and have to get to work. But this makes about as much sense as driving to the office in a car with a gas tank on empty. We would never even attempt that because if the car ran out of gas it would create a huge problem that would slow us down. Instead, we take the extra few minutes required to fill the tank so that we are sure we have enough fuel to get to the office.

Skipping breakfast is no different. If several hours have passed since you awoke before you have eaten anything, you are severely slowing down your metabolism and hindering your weight loss efforts. Eating nothing in the morning tells your body that it needs to keep your metabolism at a slow level because it has no fuel to burn. By eating something, preferably a healthy, hearty full breakfast, you jump start your metabolism and give it something to burn, in effect cranking it up for the rest of the day.

Not only is it important to eat something for breakfast, it is important to eat the right things. Like all our other meals, a good breakfast should include protein, a moderate amount of carbohydrates and a small amount of fat. An example of a healthy breakfast would be two egg whites with one yolk, a serving of Kashi Go Lean cereal with skim milk, and a cup of coffee with nonfat creamer.

Begin routinely eating a healthy breakfast like the one described and you will be taking a big step towards reaching your weight loss goal.

Get Real Diet Plan Key #5 – Cheat in Moderation

No one is able to stick to a perfectly healthy eating plan all the time. My personal weakness is sweets. After you reach your target weight and shift to a maintenance program it is certainly acceptable to indulge your craving in moderation.

However, while you are working on losing weight and reaching your goal, you should avoid or at least limit as much as possible how often and how much you cheat. By following the Get Real Plan you should find yourself having far fewer cravings because it is such a balanced eating plan, but knowing that it is difficult for most people to go for weeks at a time without an occasional lapse, let me give you some good cheats that you use when you have a weak moment. The following cheats are to be used in moderation, meaning one to two times per week only:

- 1 to 2 ounces full-fat cheese
- all natural peanut, almond, or cashew butter (in addition to the three to four serving per week allowance)
- fat-free popcorn
- reduced fat ice cream (one serving) – ideally, sugar-free as well
- red wine (1 glass)
- light beer (1 can or bottle)

Another rule of thumb when you really want to cheat on any food is my "three bite rule." If you're presented with your favorite dish or dessert, take three bites, enjoy them, and then call it quits.

Also, here are a few foods that are actually not cheats, even though they may seem like a treat to you. Incorporate them into your meals as a guilt-free indulgence. They include:

- sugar-free jello
- light or plain yogurt (make sure it is one with 10 grams of sugar per serving maximum)
- rice cakes spread with low fat cream cheese or peanut butter
- pickles (be aware of the high sodium, which is bad for water retention)
- Kashi granola bars
- Kashi crackers (or other whole grain crackers) with hummus, cheese, or peanut butter

Get Real Diet Plan Strategy #6 – Eat the Right Proportion of Protein, Carbs, & Fat at Each Meal

While most people who eat poorly know that their diet is bad, they do not know why it is bad and exactly what they should do differently. Let's dissect a typical junk food meal by picking on an American icon, McDonald's. A common meal would include a Quarter Pounder with cheese, medium french fries, and a 12-ounce coke.

Everyone knows this meal is bad for you, but can you guess what is out of balance about it? Aside from the fact that it is extremely high in calories and has way too much sugar (Coke is basically liquefied sugar), the proportions between the carbs, fat, and protein are way out of whack.

This meal contains a huge amount of fat, thanks to the high-fat cheese, french fries, and high-fat hamburger meat. It also contains an enormous amount of carbohydrates from the french fries, Coke, and the white bread bun. While it does have some protein from the hamburger meat, it is not much, especially when you consider the total amount of calories contained in the meal.

Here is the damage: 1,030 calories, 127 grams of carbohydrates, 45 grams of fat, and only 33 grams of protein. And I didn't even Supersize it! As explained above, the proper balance between the three food categories (carbs, protein, and fat) helps your body to increase your metabolism and more effectively burn calories. Obviously, this kind of meal needs to be avoided and replaced with a Get Real Meal. Here is a chart to give you an overall idea of what you should be consuming at each of the five daily meals.

Get Real Diet Plan Daily Meal Chart

Below is a chart to give you an overall idea of what you should consume at each of the five daily meals. As I will explain later, the amount of servings may need to be adjusted if you experience a lot of hunger, but the proportions should remain consistent.

BREAKFAST:

1 serving carbohydrate
1 serving protein
1 serving dairy (optional)

MID-MORNING SNACK:

1 serving fruit with 1 serving protein, or
1 serving carbohydrate with 1 serving protein

LUNCH:

1 serving non-refined carbohydrate
1 serving protein
2 servings vegetables

MID-AFTERNOON SNACK:

1 serving fruit with 1 serving protein, or
1 serving complex carbohydrate with 1 serving protein

DINNER:

1 serving protein
3 servings vegetables

Get Real Diet Plan Sample Menus

The Daily Meal Chart shown on the previous page gives you the basic outline needed in order to create your meals, Get Real style. But to make it super simple and get you off to a fast start, starting on the next page you will find a week's worth of sample menus. I really recommend that you get creative and begin planning your own meals that fit your personal preferences. This will help you to avoid boredom and monotony with the same foods repeated over and over, but for now these menus will give you a good starting point.

Get Real Sample Menu - Day One

BREAKFAST:

English muffin (whole grain)
egg white omelet (two eggs)
one slice low-fat cheese

MID-MORNING SNACK:

Kashi Bar with peanut butter

LUNCH:

grilled chicken breast with salad
fruit

MID-AFTERNOON SNACK:

nonfat plain Greek yogurt with berries

DINNER:

grilled salmon
grilled vegetables (two servings)
side salad

Get Real Sample Menu - Day Two

BREAKFAST:

Kashi Go-Lean cereal (add flax seed)
Skim milk

MID-MORNING SNACK:

apple
low-fat cheese

LUNCH:

grilled chicken sandwich (with light
wheat bread)

MID-AFTERNOON SNACK:

whole grain crackers with hummus

DINNER:

turkey burger
steamed vegetables (two servings)
side salad

Get Real Sample Menu - Day Three

BREAKFAST:

oatmeal
egg white omelet

MID-MORNING SNACK:

whey protein smoothie (made with whey
protein powder, berries, sweetener, and
water)

LUNCH:

chicken fajitas (with salsa and
guacamole) with one corn tortilla or rice
or beans

MID-AFTERNOON SNACK:

yogurt

DINNER:

baked tilapia
vegetables (two servings)
side salad

Get Real Sample Menu - Day Four

BREAKFAST:

whole grain toast with peanut butter
skim milk

MID-MORNING SNACK:

peach
low-fat cottage cheese

LUNCH:

lean hamburger with ½ whole wheat
bun
salad

MID-AFTERNOON SNACK:

hummus with celery

DINNER:

chicken with mushrooms
spinach (two servings)
side salad

Get Real Sample Menu - Day Five

BREAKFAST:

whole grain toast with low-sugar jam
low-fat cottage cheese

MID-MORNING SNACK:

apple with peanut butter

LUNCH:

scrambled eggs with vegetables in whole
grain tortilla wrap with low fat cheese

MID-AFTERNOON SNACK:

Greek yogurt with berries

DINNER:

turkey meatloaf
side salad
grilled vegetables (one or two servings)

Get Real Sample Menu - Day Six

BREAKFAST:

oatmeal
egg whites

MID-MORNING SNACK:

whey protein shake (protein & water only)
Kashi bar

LUNCH:

shrimp salad
pear

MID-AFTERNOON SNACK:

whole wheat toast with low-fat cheese

DINNER:

grilled snapper with lump crabmeat
grilled vegetables

Get Real Sample Menu - Day Seven

BREAKFAST:

cottage cheese with berries

MID-MORNING SNACK:

yogurt

LUNCH:

pasta (whole wheat) with grilled chicken
and vegetables

MID-AFTERNOON SNACK:

whole grain crackers and low-fat cheese

DINNER:

tofu or chicken stir fry with vegetables

Protein and Carb Serving Sizes

In order to follow the Get Real Diet Plan you need a basic understanding of serving sizes. While this may seem cumbersome at first, it will become second nature for you in no time.

The following charts contain serving sizes for some common carbohydrates and proteins.

Carbohydrates:	Serving Size
dry cereal	3/4 -1 cup
oatmeal	½ cup (cooked)
bread	One slice
lentils (kidney, black, pinto beans)	½ cup cooked
English muffin	½ muffin
bagel	¼ to ½ bagel
hot dog or hamburger bun	½ bun
potatoes	1 medium
butternut squash	1 cup
corn tortillas	1 tortilla
corn	½ cup or 1 ear
carrots	½ cup or 1 carrot
cream of wheat	½ cup cooked
peas	½ cup
rice (preferably brown or wild)	½ cup cooked
pasta	½ cup cooked

Carbohydrates:	Serving Size
high fiber cereal (Fiber One or Kashi Go Lean)	¾ cup to 1 cup
yogurt (reduced or fat-free)	1 cup
fruits	1 med. size pc.
fat free/skim milk	1 cup

Proteins:	Serving Size
boneless, skinless chicken breast	3 oz.
boneless, skinless turkey breast	3 oz.
ground turkey breast (97-99% lean)	3 oz.
fish	3 to 4 oz.
tuna (in water, not oil)	3 to 4 oz.
lean beef (93% or leaner)	3 oz.
veal	3 oz.
cottage cheese (2% fat or less)	½ cup
reduced fat natural cheeses (Swiss, cheddar, mozzarella)	1½ oz
reduced fat processed cheese (American)	2 oz.
egg whites (not yolk)	3-4 eggs
egg substitute	½ cup

Proteins:	Serving Size
tofu	3-4 oz or ½ c
egg, whole	1

For additional serving sizes please refer to the appendix. For foods not listed above or in the appendix, use the serving size listed on the food labels.

What If You Follow The Plan But Find You Are Still Hungry?

It is important to understand that the amount of calories a person requires varies depending on a number of factors, as mentioned earlier.

So if you follow the program and frequently find yourself very hungry, then you probably need to add more calories into your diet. You should do this is by proportionately increasing your portions slightly, thus keeping your ratio of carbohydrates, protein and fat consistent with the program guidelines.

What you should not do is pick and choose what you want to eliminate. For instance, if you feel breakfast is too much food, you should not eat only the carbohydrate and skip the protein. Similarly, you should not make substitutions, like at dinner replacing the protein with a carbohydrate.

Here is an example of the correct way to alter the diet. Let's say you find yourself consistently still somewhat hungry after lunch. Instead of having one serving of protein and one serving of carb at lunch, increase it to 1 ½ servings of each. This will help you to meet your body's caloric needs while retaining the metabolic advantages of a balanced meal.

After you make a diet change of this sort, pay attention to your results and how you feel. If you have issues like this with more than one meal, or if you find yourself getting too full (a common complaint when people begin eating five meals a day), you can make similar modifications. Just make sure that the ratios stay consistent.

It is important to avoid arbitrarily adding or eliminating foods from the diet or changing the sizes of the meals. The program is designed to provide a well balanced dietary intake of foods and altering the ratios will reduce the benefits you receive. For example, many people are in the habit of eating little to no breakfast and then having lunch and dinner that are far too big. If this is you, you may find sticking with the balanced five meals a challenge at first, but stick with it and you will very quickly start to feel a lot better, not to mention you will begin to lose weight.

Another adjustment you can make if you feel like you are not getting sufficiently full is to add additional servings of vegetables. Remember, they are considered a "free" food (other than the exceptions mentioned) and you can add as many servings of them as you like.

Chapter 10

Restaurant Guide, Shopping List & a Few Get Real Kitchen Tips

In the past you may have encountered a lot of trouble with stocking your refrigerator and pantry. It is very easy to "fall off the wagon" when we have the wrong foods around and hunger pains strike. To avoid this kind of temptation in the future I have created a detailed shopping list so you can stay properly stocked up with the right foods.

Based on this eating program, you know you need to have fresh fruits and vegetables, lean proteins, and complex carbohydrates as your main staple foods. Depending on your weaknesses, you might also want to select a few of the "good cheats" from the list provided in Chapter Nine.

If you are someone who has a tough time saying no to temptation, you should do your best to avoid having those junk foods at home that you find most appealing. Remember, while the Get Real Diet allows you to cheat occasionally, you should not exceed the maximum of one or two cheats per week. For example don't buy a large container of ice cream if you know that you will have a really hard time limiting yourself to just those two servings per week and instead you might eat the whole carton at one sitting.

Also, if you have a hard time getting satisfied by a small amount of a cheat and instead find yourself going overboard, then you might find it beneficial to avoid cheating altogether. The important thing is to know your behavior patterns and make adjustments that will help you to succeed. You can do it! No more sabotaging your efforts!

Get Real Sample Grocery List

FRUITS:

- apples
- kiwi
- berries
- oranges

VEGETABLES:

- lettuce
- cucumber
- tomatoes
- green beans
- broccoli
- spinach
- bell peppers
- zucchini

COMPLEX CARBOHYDRATES:

- oats
- sugar-free whole wheat bread
- sweet potatoes
- brown rice
- corn tortillas or low-carb or whole wheat tortillas
- high fiber cereal
- yogurt
- skim milk

LEAN PROTEINS:

- skinless chicken breasts
- lean ground turkey
- shrimp/fish
- lean beef
- cottage cheese (red. fat)

- eggs
- Greek yogurt

CHEATS:

- light ice cream
- popcorn

Get Real Grocery Shopping Tips

Your shopping can become really simple if you break it down into the five categories listed above. Give some thought to what you will be eating for the week and you will be well on your way to a successful shopping trip. For example, if you plan on eating two fruits per day you will need to buy 14 pieces of fruit, assuming you plan on shopping only once that week. Since your non-starchy vegetable intake is unlimited you will want to buy a sufficient variety of vegetables you like. Remember to choose from fresh or frozen vegetables, not canned. After a few weeks you will get used to shopping this way and it will become easier than ever.

There is one very important final issue that we need to address. You need to get rid of all the food that is not on the Get Real Plan so you are not constantly tempted by it. If this food is still going to be eaten by your spouse or children, then you need to physically separate it from your food. This may seem like overkill, but it is not. You need to have an area of the pantry and refrigerator that is exclusively for you and is without temptation. Trust me on this, it will be a lot easier for you to avoid temptation if you have your own area that has only healthy foods. Just know where your pitfalls lie, so you are best able to avoid them.

Dining Out the Get Real Way

Now that we have covered how to shop and eat at home, let's discuss eating out at restaurants. Restaurant meals are usually loaded with excess calories and fat, so when dining out you must be extremely careful what you order.

You also want to avoid eating out excessively because it is more difficult to stay on the plan while eating at restaurants. Let's face it, restaurants are temptation landmines. While it is a lot easier to control what you eat when you are preparing the food yourself, you may not like to cook or know how, you may travel a lot, you may have to frequently entertain clients, or you may simply not have the time to cook. If you fall into one of these categories, then you need to get a bit more creative (refer to Chapter 2) and just be very particular about what you eat when dining out.

I will break down the good and bad choices for restaurants based on the ethnicity of the food.

American Restaurants

Let's start with good old American cuisine. Many of the suggestions I make here are applicable to other types of food as well. Your best bet with American food would be some kind of lean protein with grilled or steamed vegetables, or a salad with grilled meat or fish on top, and this can be supplemented with a small carbohydrate.

When ordering your protein the things to avoid are: heavy sauces on top, added butter and oil, and, of course, anything fried. So when ordering your protein ask for the sauce on the side (if it comes with one) and then you can sprinkle it on your entree versus drowning it. Done this way you get the flavor without adding too much of the fat or calories. Additionally, ask them to prepare your protein without using butter or oil. While some restaurants don't saturate the food with this added fat, most do.

Another favorite at American restaurants is the basic sandwich. Here you need to be careful of the type of bread they use. If it is not whole grain (most likely it will not be) you should cut the bread consumption to half. Also pay attention to what is in your sandwich. For example, a tuna or chicken salad sandwich might sound healthy, but most of the time it is not. Most restaurants use full fat mayonnaise, so these sandwiches are loaded with fat and calories. Also, avoid having too much cheese on the sandwich because the restaurant is almost certain to use the full-fat variety.

Finally, let's talk about salad pitfalls. The biggest problem here is the salad dressing. Believe it or not, the salad dressing on your salad can have an amount of fat equivalent to a hamburger! So you want to order a low fat dressing on the side. If the restaurant does not have that as an option then you should order oil and vinegar on the side. You want to sprinkle the oil sparingly and use more vinegar. If you can handle your salad with very little dressing you can get the full fat one and use it very sparingly, just to get the flavor. Other hidden fat on salads are croutons, bacon, and lots of cheese. These should be avoided altogether.

All this modifying might seem overly complicated or excessive to you at first, but it really makes a major difference nutritionally and helps you to avoid taking a step backward every time you eat out. It will very quickly become second nature for you to order your food according to your specifications. After all, you're paying for it so why not get it the way you want?

Italian Restaurants

Let's move on to Italian food. Here the biggest pitfalls are the carbohydrates. You can't have all that pasta! Now, you can have some on the side but it cannot consume most of your entree. You also need to be careful with the sauces at Italian restaurants. Your best choice is a tomato-based sauce, not an Alfredo or other cream-based sauce. For instance, a Marsala sauce is a better choice than a wine and butter sauce. Just like the American restaurants, you should ask that your food be prepared without butter or oil. Another thing you want to avoid is breading on your protein. It is not the worst thing, but some places overdo it. If you do order something that has a lot of breading, then consider that as your carbohydrate. Just remember, you want a good lean protein on your plate and some vegetables.

Here's a pointer that works well in an Italian restaurant. How do you know there's too much oil or butter in the food you're eating? When you rub your lips together and you can feel the grease, that is definitely too much fat!

Another issue to watch for in Italian restaurants is the bread. Most Italian restaurants automatically bring it to your table, which is a temptation you do not need. The best way to handle this is to simply ask your waiter to take it away from the table. If you do eat the bread, then have just one piece and consider that your carb for the meal. Also, make sure you use the butter or olive oil sparingly with your bread.

Mexican Restaurants

Next is Mexican food. Again, many of the previously mentioned guidelines will apply here. With Mexican food, you need to be especially careful of the tortillas. Most restaurants have flour tortillas made with lard or fat. A much better choice is the corn tortillas. And of course, you have to avoid the tortilla chips. Just ask the waiter not to bring them to your table.

As you know, Mexican food is heavy on the cheeses so you should ask for your food to be prepared "light on the cheese." Even better would be ordering fajitas without the skin (if chicken) and without any butter glaze (yes, they usually top it off with more fat).

You could eat one or two corn tortillas and have more protein (for example, chicken) on the side. You can sprinkle it with a little cheese, but avoid the sour cream. Also, your freebie here is the salsa and pico de gallo. No hidden fat there! As you might recall, guacamole (made from avocados) does contain good fat, but fat nonetheless. Therefore, have a spoonful and leave it at that.

Again, you should be careful with your choices of sauces. Stick to the red, tomato-based sauce and avoid cream-based sauces, such as creamy cilantro. One more thing to note, refried beans, black beans, and charro beans are all good for you but they are carbohydrates. Consequently, if you're eating tortillas, you've filled your carbohydrate quota and you should not have the beans. By now you are probably starting to notice the trend of how we want to balance the protein, carbohydrates, and fat at each meal.

Chinese and Thai Restaurants

Now let's discuss some Asian foods like Chinese and Thai. These foods can be healthy because many of the entrees consist of protein and vegetables, but the most common problem with Asian food is when it is stir fried with too much oil. While you are trying to lose weight you just can't afford high fat consumption.

Your best choices at most Chinese or Thai restaurants will be the steamed dishes. It is important to note that many dishes not listed on the menu as steamed can be requested as steamed.

While you will want to avoid egg rolls, you can have the non-fried spring rolls. You will also want to watch your rice consumption and remember to refer to the index for serving sizes. Stick to steamed white or brown rice, not fried rice or noodles.

Japanese Restaurants

In the Japanese category, we have sushi and sashimi. Some of the better low-fat choices are rolls made with fish, shrimp, crab, or vegetables. Make sure you have them prepared without the mayonnaise and cream cheese. Just pay attention to the ingredients and don't be afraid to ask your waiter questions about what the dishes contain.

Sashimi is also a good choice, as you get the fish without the other things (including rice) added to it. Other low fat choices for sushi and sashimi include cod, snapper, tilapia, scallops, shrimp, and flounder, to name a few.

Seafood Restaurants

Now let's move on to seafood restaurants. Yes, you will see many fried choices, but you need to stick to the grilled fish. Again, ask for it to be cooked without oil and butter. Have a salad and/or steamed or grilled vegetables on the side with half a potato.

Breakfast and Brunch

Lastly, let's talk about having breakfast or brunch at a restaurant. Your best choice for protein would be an egg white or egg substitute omelet with vegetables (optional). Your best choice of a carbohydrate would be oatmeal. The oatmeal should be ordered without added sugar, butter or cream. You can sweeten it with your sweetener of choice and cinnamon.

Pastries should be avoided because of excessive sugar and fat. If you really want pancakes or waffles, limit it to one and use sugar-free syrup without butter on top. Avoid bacon and sausage as your proteins because of the excessive fat.

These are all suggestions to make your life easier while sticking to the plan when dining out. If you really feel the need to cheat while dining out, just remember to limit your quantity. It is okay, we all cheat some of the time. The difference is how often we cheat and how much we eat when we cheat. Just remember, portion sizes really do matter.

A Few Get Real Diet Kitchen Tips

The following are some tips for use in the kitchen.

Canola & Olive Oil Instead Of Butter – Use olive or canola oil (sparingly) and fat free cooking spray as a substitute for butter. This will help lower your intake of saturated fat.

Measure With a Scale at First – At first you will want to measure out the quantities so you can get familiar with what an appropriate serving size looks like. You will be surprised at how small a half cup or a full cup actually is.

Foods to Avoid and Get Real Substitutes

We have discussed in great detail what you should eat, but we should also talk about some common food and drinks to avoid. These items contain a lot of hidden fat and calories that may inhibit weight loss. Where appropriate, I have suggested healthier alternatives.

1. Coffee Drinks

Regular "drip" coffee is fine, just make sure you use skim milk instead of cream. The real problem at coffee houses like Starbucks is the very popular blended drinks that are full of fat and sugar. See the appendix for Starbucks nutritional values and you will probably be shocked by the amount of calories and fat you are getting with that mocha frappaccino with whipped cream.

Good choices: non-fat latte, non-fat cappuccino, unsweetened iced coffee. You can sweeten your drinks with Splenda or other artificial sweeteners.

Bad choices: full fat latte or cappuccino, seasonal lattes (pumpkin, peppermint, etc.), frappaccinos, mocha and caramel drinks with whipped cream.

2. Smoothies (store bought)

Most smoothies made at specialty stores contain a lot of calories from both the sugar content in the fruit, as well as additional sugar that is added.

Good choice: make at home with whey protein powder, fruit (fresh or frozen), water and/or skim milk, light yogurt, and sweetener (optional).

3. Fat-Free Foods

Fat-free foods often have higher sugar content. Remember, that translates to a quicker surge in blood sugar and insulin levels.

4. Some Misc. Foods & Drinks to Avoid

The following are generally unhealthy and should be avoided:

- cream based sauces (alfredo, creamy tomato, etc.)
- cream based soups (chowders and cream of chicken, mushroom, etc.)
- dips
- sour cream, full-fat – reduced fat or fat-free are good substitutes
- salad dressings – reduced fat or fat-free are good substitutes, but beware of the sugar content
- croutons
- mayonnaise – fat-free or light are acceptable
- sandwich spreads
- most granola and fruit bars
- sodas (contain 150 calories with seven or more teaspoons of sugar in a 12 ounce serving!) – one to two diet sodas a day are allowed
- fruit juices (contain similar amount of calories as the soda) – sugar-free drinks such as Crystal Light are allowed
- sweetened tea – unsweetened is allowed
- creamers – fat-free and unsweetened are allowed
- alcohol

Part Four –

Conclusion

Chapter 11

Parting Words –
The Reality of Weight Loss

Unlike a lot of plans that make false "easy weight loss" promises, the Get Real promise is that you can absolutely achieve your weight loss goals if you are committed to doing the work and following the plan.

While there are plenty of magic pills advertised that claim you can eat anything you want and still lose weight, the reality is that you need to change your lifestyle if you want to maintain a healthy weight. This plan may seem daunting at first because anything different than maintaining the status quo will seem difficult. But compare this to a promotion you might get offered at work for a position with more responsibilities and higher pay. You might be a little nervous about it, but you would take the challenge because of your desire to reap the benefits.

Endeavoring into this new eating and exercise plan is no different. It is something you are not comfortable with because it is new and different. But as you incorporate the plan into your life you will find that it will replace the old status quo and these activities that seem difficult at the beginning will become part of your daily habits. Eventually, you will wonder why you ever had such bad, unhealthy habits to begin with and you will become a full-blown convert to a more enjoyable, healthier lifestyle.

The Importance of Accountability

One of the big keys to getting through this initial stage and creating good habits is using accountability to help keep you on track. Just like having a manager at the workplace who keeps you accountable for doing your job properly, you really need someone who can help keep you accountable on your weight loss project. This can be in the form of hiring a personal trainer, nutritionist, exercise partner, or getting your spouse or even the whole family involved.

Make sure that you do not underestimate the importance of accountability. This is probably the most common reason that people fail to reach their weight loss goals. Lack of accountability makes it so much easier to give in when you have a craving or are feeling lazy. I want you to successfully tackle your weight loss goal this time and that requires accountability.

Consider how many celebrities seem to get in great shape successfully. Why are they able to do it with seeming ease when the rest of us struggle? The difference is that they have a great support network. If you had similar support you would get similar results! So make sure you take advantage of a support system to help propel you towards your goal.

This is especially helpful when you have the same trouble areas that pop up again and again. For instance, if you have a history of intending to go to the gym but never actually making it, this is a perfect area to use your support system. You could get a workout partner and agree to a workout schedule together. With someone counting on you to meet them there it will be a lot harder to skip. Or you could write down your exercise schedule and then give it to a friend or family member with the agreement that you will go over your results with them once a week. Knowing that you are going to have to admit that you did not live up to your schedule will give you some added incentive to get to the gym.

The option most likely to help you reach your goal is to hire a good personal trainer. While many people consider a personal trainer an unnecessary expense you really have to ask yourself how important your health is and how much it is worth to you to finally get in the shape you want to achieve. Also, many trainers offer group sessions with two to five clients at reduced rates. So if you have a friend who is trying to get in shape also you can team up and get the benefits of a trainer at a reduced cost.

If it still seems too expensive, then you might want to take a closer look at how you spend your money and consider reallocating your funds. Depending on how much you spend on eating out, drinking, shopping, and other luxuries you might be able to cut back so that you have some funds available.

I am dwelling on the point of exercise because I know that this is the biggest challenge for many people. Having been a personal trainer for over a decade I know that most people have hang ups about getting to the gym and are capable of coming up with all kinds of creative excuses to avoid it. Having a trainer can make your workouts not just more effective, but actually enjoyable.

My clients always mention how the time goes by so much faster when they are working out with me. And believe me, it's not because they're not working hard!

You can do this! No matter which method you choose you can get consistent about exercise. You can go for walks, use exercise videos at home, take up a sport you haven't played in years, or go to the gym. Remember, it is all about moving. It is the way our bodies were intended to function.

Let's talk a little bit more about accountability, this time as it relates to the eating plan. If you are single then you have total control over your pantry and refrigerator and can eliminate all temptations from your kitchen. You also can make arrangements with friends according to your needs. Remember, you can order food at almost any restaurant to your specifications.

If you are married or have children, you will probably have to exercise some will power in avoiding temptations, but it can be done. Ideally, you will get your spouse onboard and have them as your partner in the program. To make things fun, if one of you reaches a predetermined goal, the other person has to give them a reward of their choice. There is nothing wrong with creating incentives! It is all about getting and staying motivated. If it is not possible for your spouse to partake in the program with you, then just make sure to explain how important this project is to you and that you really need their support.

This is Not a Quick-Fix Plan

As you begin your weight loss journey remember that success will come in baby steps. The Get Real program is not about seeing how fast you can get there, it is about achieving real, healthy, lasting results.

Our culture is constantly bombarded with outlandish messages preying on people's desire to get fit, while promising they can do it very quickly, with no effort, while they continue to eat anything they want in large quantities. You don't want to ever fall victim to these phony ads again.

Since I get so many questions about the latest fads that are advertised let me be completely clear about most of the diet and weight loss products out there. The advertisements claiming that you only have to take their pill, make no other lifestyle changes and the pounds will just melt away, well, those claims are bogus.

The ads that claim people dramatically altered their bodies by using a single piece of equipment a few minutes a day without making any other lifestyle changes, those are lies, too. The ads for the latest fad diet contain similar bogus claims.

The truth is that there is no easy quick fix. The truth is that reaching your target weight takes work and dedication, but it is so worth it. Fads come and fads go, but the proven fundamentals of weight loss stay the same. If you practice those fundamentals consistently you will reach your goal, guaranteed.

It is time for you to stop listening to the crowd that will try to lure you into wasting money on their false promises of easy weight loss. Remember that if it sounds too good to be true, it probably is. Deep down, we all know that weight loss requires commitment, so don't let these con artists take advantage of you.

Keep your sanity and follow this structured, real life plan. You will at times feel frustrated because it is difficult to be patient, but you are not alone. There are a lot of people just like you who have done the program, have experienced the same feelings of frustration as you will, and then come out on the other end victorious. Just keep the faith in knowing that it is normal to get a little frustrated and keep going.

Whether this is your first time or one hundredth attempt to lose weight, see it as a fresh start. I want to wish you good luck on your weight loss journey and congratulations on starting a new life as a healthier, stronger, more energized and confident you!

APPENDIX 1

FOOD NUTRITIONAL VALUES

Fruit

Food	Calories	Carbs (grams)	Fat (grams)
Apple	80	22	0
Avocado (half)	140	8	**13**
Banana	**110**	29	0
Blackberries (1 cup)	70	18	0.5
Blueberries (1 cup)	80	20	0.5
Cantaloupe (1 cup)	100	23	1
Cherries (1 cup)	90	22	0.5
Coconut (fresh, 50 grams)	**180**	8	**17**
Cranberries (1 cup)	45	12	0
Figs (fresh)	45	12	0
Grapes (1 cup)	60	16	0.5
Grapefruit (1/2 piece)	60	16	0
Honeydew (1/4 melon)	**130**	33	0
Kiwifruit	50	12	0.5
Mango	**130**	35	0.5
Nectarine	70	16	0.5

Food	Calories	Carbs (grams)	Fat (grams)
Orange	45	14	0
Papaya	**120**	30	0
Passion Fruit (3 pieces)	50	13	0
Peach	40	11	0
Pear	100	25	1
Pineapple (1 cup)	80	19	0.5
Plantain	**220**	57	0.5
Plum	40	10	0.5
Pomegranate	100	26	0
Raspberries (1 cup)	60	14	0.5
Strawberries (1 cup)	30	8	0
Tangerine	50	15	0.5
Watermelon (2 cups)	80	27	0

*all items are for medium size piece fruit, unless otherwise specified

items in **bold indicate especially high fat or calorie fruits

Vegetables

Food	Calories	Carbs (grams)
Artichokes (1 med.)	60	13
Asparagus (5 spears)	25	4
Beets	35	8
Bell Pepper (Green or Red)	30	8
Bok Choy (half head)	50	9
Broccoli (3 med. Spears)	25	5
Brussels Sprouts (5 med.)	40	9
Cabbage (Green or Red)	60	12
Carrots	35	8
Cauliflower (1/4 head)	35	7
Celery	10	3
Collard Greens (100 grams)	30	6
Corn, Sweet (1 ear)	120	27
Cucumber	45	9
Eggplant	140	33
Fennel	70	17
Garlic (2 cloves)	10	2
Ginger (15 grams)	15	4
Green Beans (100 grams)	30	6
Horseradish Root (1 Tbsp.)	10	2

Food	Calories	Carbs (grams)
Jerusalem Artichoke (100 grams)	80	17
Jicama	140	32
Kale (100 grams)	50	10
Leeks	50	13
Lettuce (Boston, Bibb, Butter) (1 head)	20	4
Lettuce (Iceberg)	45	9
Lettuce (Red or Green Leaf, 100 grams)	20	4
Lettuce (Romaine, 100 grams)	15	2
Mushrooms (Crimini) (50 grams)	10	2
Mushrooms (Shiitake) (100 grams)	25	5
Mustard Greens (100 grams)	25	5
Okra (100 grams)	35	8
Onion (Red or Yellow)	40	9
Parsley (1 cup)	20	4
Parsnip	80	18
Potato	100	26
Pumpkin (1 cup mashed)	50	12
Radish (3 pieces)	5	1
Rhubarb (1 cup)	25	6
Rutabaga	70	16
Savoy Cabbage (1 cup)	20	4
Scallion (100 grams)	30	7

Food	Calories	Carbs (grams)
Snow Peas (100 grams)	40	8
Spinach (100 grams)	20	4
Squash (Acorn)	170	45
Squash (Butternut) (1 cup)	60	16
Sweet Potato	130	33
Swiss Chard (100 grams)	20	4
Tomato	35	7
Tomato (Cherry) (5)	20	4
Tomato (Roma) (3)	40	9
Turnip	35	8
Turnip Greens (100 grams)	25	6
Zucchini	45	9

*all items are for medium size vegetable, unless otherwise specified

*One serving of raw vegetables = one cup

*One serving of cooked vegetables = 1/2 cup

*Note that the following vegetables have a higher amount of carbohydrates: artichokes, corn, eggplant, fennel, jicama, parsnip, potato, sweet potato and squash

Meat

Food	Serving Size	Calories	Fat (grams)
Chicken Breast	3 oz. (skinless)	142	5
Chicken Drumstick	2 drumsticks (roasted, no skin)	150	5
Chicken Leg (thigh & drumstick)	3 oz. (roasted, no skin)	181	5
Chicken Thighs	2 oz. (1 thigh) (roasted, no skin)	109	6
Chicken Wings	2 wings (roasted no skin)	85	4
Duck	3 oz. (roasted)	170	12
Goose	3 oz. (roasted)	202	11
Turkey (white meat)	3 oz. (roasted)	135	2
Turkey (dark meat)	3 oz. (roasted)	159	4
Buffalo/Bison	3 oz.	130	2
Beef brisket	3 oz.	206	11
Beef ribs	3 oz.	190	10
Eye Round Roast	3 oz.	140	3

Food	Serving Size	Calories	Fat (grams)
Top Round Sirloin	3 oz.	153	5
Beef Tenderloin	3 oz.	170	7
Porterhouse Steak	3 oz.	185	9
Beef, Ground (95% lean)	3 oz.	127	5
Beef, Ground (90% lean)	3 oz.	164	9
Beef, Ground (80% lean)	3 oz.	231	16
Pork Tenderloin	3 oz.	140	4
Pork Sirloin Chop	3 oz.	165	6
Pork Loin Chop	3 oz.	171	7
Pork Ribs	3 oz.	210	13
Bacon (cooked)	2 slices	88	7
Canadian Bacon	2 slices	88	4
Ham			
Lamb (varies based on cut)	3 oz.	175-300	8-16
Goat	3 oz.	122	2.6

*All values are approximations

Seafood

Food	Calories	Protein (grams)	Fat (grams)
Blue Crab	90	19	1
Catfish	120	19	5
Clam	130	22	2
Cod	90	19	1
Flounder	100	20	1
Haddock	90	20	1
Halibut	120	22	2
Lobster	100	20	1
Mackerel	190	21	12
Mahi Mahi	90	20	1
Ocean Perch	100	20	2
Orange Roughy	70	16	1
Oyster	120	12	4
Pollock	100	21	1
Rainbow Trout	130	22	4
Rockfish	100	20	2
Salmon (Atlantic)	150	22	5
Salmon (Sockeye Red)	190	24	9.5
Scallops (6 large or 14 small)	150	29	1
Shrimp	110	22	2
Sole	100	21	1
Swordfish	130	21	4
Tilapia	100	21	1

Food	Calories	Protein (grams)	Fat (grams)
Tuna	120	25	1

*All values based on 3 ounce serving size of fish prepared by baking or grilling.

Healthy Fats

Food	Serving Size	Calories	Protein (g)	Fat (g)
Flaxseed (whole)	1 Tsp.	18.2	0.6	1.4
Flaxseed (ground)	1 Tsp.	13.4	0.5	1.1
Flaxseed Oil	1 Tbsp.	120	0	13.6
Olives	6 olives	50	0	5
Almonds	1 oz. (22 almonds)	160	6	14
Brazil Nuts	1 oz. (7 nuts)	190	4	19
Cashews	1 oz. (16-18 nuts)	160	4	13
Hazelnuts	1 oz. (18-20 nuts)	180	4	17
Macadamias	1 oz. (10-12 nuts)	200	2	22
Peanuts	1 oz. (28 nuts)	170	7	14
Pecans	1 oz. (18-20 halves)	200	3	20
Pine nuts	1 oz. (150-157 nuts)	160	7	14
Pistachios	1 oz. (45-47 nuts)	160	6	13
Walnuts	1 oz. (14 halves)	190	4	18

Alcohol

Beverage	Serving Size	Calories (Avg.)
Beer, regular	12 oz.	149
Beer, light	12 oz.	110
Gin, rum, vodka, whisky, tequila	1 oz.	65
Brandy, cognac	1 oz.	65
Liqueurs (Cointreau, Kahlua)	1.5 oz.	188
Red Wine	4 oz.	80
Dry White Wine	4 oz.	75
Sweet Wine	4 oz.	105
Sherry Wine	2 oz.	75
Port Wine	2 oz.	90
Champagne	4 oz.	84
Vermouth, sweet	3 oz.	140
Vermouth, dry	3 oz.	105

APPENDIX 2

RESTAURANT NUTRITIONAL VALUES

Fast Food Restaurant: Chick-Fil-A

Food	Calories	Carb (g)	Sugar (g)	Protein (g)	Fat (g)
Chargrilled chicken club sandwich	370	34	9	35	11
Chargrilled chicken sandwich *	260	33	9	27	3
Chick-n-Strips	260	33	9	27	3
Chicken Salad Sandwich	500	53	13	29	20
Chicken Sandwich	410	39	5	27	16
Nuggets	410	39	5	27	16
Bacon, Egg & Cheese Biscuit	440	34	5	19	26
Biscuit	240	33	4	4	11
Biscuit & Gravy	360	44	5	8	17
Chick-n-Minis	360	44	5	8	17

Food	Calories	Carb (g)	Sugar (g)	Protein (g)	Fat (g)
Chicken Biscuit	390	39	5	18	18
Chicken Breakfast Burrito	410	40	3	22	18
Chicken Egg & Cheese Bagel	500	49	8	31	20
Hash Browns	260	25	0	2	17
Sausage Biscuit	530	33	5	17	36
Sausage Breakfast Burrito	460	38	3	21	25
Barbecue Sauce	45	11	9	0	0
Blue Cheese Dressing	150	1	1	1	16
Buffalo Sauce **	10	1	0	0	0
Buttermilk Ranch Dressing	160	1	1	0	17
Buttermilk Ranch Sauce	110	1	1	0	12
Caesar Dressing	160	1	0	1	17
Chick-fil-A Sauce	140	6	6	0	13

Food	Calories	Carb (g)	Sugar (g)	Protein (g)	Fat (g)
Fat Free Honey Mustard	60	14	11	0	0
Honey Mustard Sauce	45	10	10	0	0
Honey Roasted BBQ Sauce **	60	2	2	0	5
Light Italian Dressing **	15	2	2	0	0.5
Polynesian Sauce	110	13	13	0	6
Reduced Fat Berry Balsamic Vinaigrette	70	12	9	0	2
Spicy Dressing	140	2	1	0	14
Thousand Island Dressing	150	5	4	0	14
Chargrilled & Fruit Salad **	220	20	14	22	6
Chargrilled Chicken Garden Salad **	180	10	5	23	6
Chick-n-Strips Salad	450	25	7	39	22

Food	Calories	Carb (g)	Sugar (g)	Protein (g)	Fat (g)
Garlic and Butter Croutons **	60	9	1	2	2
Harvest Nut Granola **	60	10	3	1	2
Honey Roasted Sunflower-Kernels **	90	4	1	2	7
Southwest Chargrilled Salad **	240	17	6	25	9
Tortilla Strips *	80	8	1	1	4
Chargrilled Chicken Cool Wrap	410	49	7	33	12
Chicken Caesar Cool Wrap	480	45	5	40	16
Spicy Chicken Cool Wrap	410	47	5	35	12

Note that wraps are high in carbs.

*Good Choice
**Best Choice

Bar & Grill Restaurant: Chili's

Food	Calories	Carb (g)	Protein (g)	Fat (g)
Southwestern Eggrolls w/ Avocado Ranch	910	73	27	57
Skillet Queso w/ chips	940	42	32	77
Triple Dipper Boneless Sweet Chile Glazed Wings w/ Ranch	730	49	30	45
Classic Nachos w/ Fajita Beef no guac	1550	69	90	105
Hot Spinach & Artichoke Dip w/chips	930	39	24	77
Boneless Sweet Chile Glazed Wings w/ Ranch	1250	96	56	70
Boneless Buffalo Chicken Salad	1070	46	44	78
Caesar Salad w/ Grilled Chicken	930	28	43	71
Southwestern Cobb Salad	1090	57	54	71
Side Salad House no dressing *	210	17	10	12

Food	Calories	Carb (g)	Protein (g)	Fat (g)
Baked Potato	510	26	17	35
Broccoli Cheese Soup (bowl)	250	18	11	16
Chicken Noodle Soup (bowl) **	50	18	6	1
Chicken Tortilla Soup (bowl) *	260	20	14	15
New England Clam Chowder (bowl)	370	23	12	26
Southwestern Vegetable Soup (bowl) *	210	26	9	8
Smoked Turkey Sandwich	870	75	40	48
Grilled Chicken Sandwich	810	57	46	43
Fajita Pita Chicken	380	39	30	12
Bacon Burger	1050	53	55	68
Oldtimer w/ cheese	850	55	47	48
Guiltless Carne Asada Steak **	371	11	46	10
Guiltless Buffalo Sandwich *	386	46	36	7
Guiltless Grilled Chicken Sandwich *	361	44	36	5

Food	Calories	Carb (g)	Protein (g)	Fat (g)
Guiltless Cedar Plank Tilapia **	199	8	34	4
Guiltless Honey-Mustard Glazed Salmon **	416	13	50	20
Guiltless Chicken Platter *	371	49	39	2
Classic Steak Fajitas	470	25	45	25
Classic Chicken Fajitas*	370	25	39	11
Fajita Quesadillas Beef w/ rice & beans	1580	172	79	62
Original Ribs	990	33	57	68
Honey BBQ Ribs	1120	66	57	68
Cajun Chicken Pasta	1260	93	62	67
Margarita Grilled Chicken	720	92	54	14
Chicken Club Tacos (2)	1220	122	51	58
Flame-Grilled Ribeye	1070	18	42	92
Add Rice and Kettle Black Beans*	350	73	12	2

Food	Calories	Carb (g)	Protein (g)	Fat (g)
Add Spicy & Garlic Shrimp to any Entrée **	70	1	6	4.5
Dressing, Avocado Ranch	110	2	1	11
Dressing, Bleu Cheese	240	1	1	25
Dressing, Caesar	260	2	2	27
Dressing, Honey Mustard no Fat *	70	11	0	0
Dressing, Low Fat Ranch **	45	4	1	3
Dressing, Low Fat Vinaigrette **	60	8	0	2
Homestyle Fries	430	43	4	26
Kettle Black Beans **	110	20	6	1
Seasonal Veggies **	70	7	3	4.5
Steamed Broccoli **	70	7	3	5
Cheesecake	700	67	12	42
Chocolate Chip Paradise Pie	1590	220	19	76
Molten Chocolate Cake	1290	174	13	62

Food	Calories	Carb (g)	Protein (g)	Fat (g)
Sweet Shot Double Chocolate Fudge Brownie	420	51	1	24

*Good choice
**Best choice

Italian Restaurant: Macaroni Grill

Food	Calories	Carb (g)	Protein (g)	Fat (g)
Chicken Caesar Salad	870	31	42	67
Insalata Blu w/chicken	780	19	45	56
Mozzarella Alla Caprese (3)	250	5	11	21
Parmesan-Crusted Chicken	1100	66	83	58
Warm Spinach Salad	510	20	19	43
Chicken Toscana (1 bowl)	540	42	24	31
Tomato Basil with Cheese Tortellini (1 bowl)	520	79	27	11
Calamari Fritti	1180	65	43	81
Crab-Stuffed Mushrooms	590	41	29	36
Shrimp & Artichoke Dip	910	86	33	49
Tomato Bruschetta	990	78	18	67
Sizzling Shrimp Scampi	1500	94	49	100

Food	Calories	Carb (g)	Protein (g)	Fat (g)
Chicken & Shrimp Scaloppine, Dinner	1510	68	64	113
Chicken Cannelloni, Dinner	880	61	59	44
Chicken Marsala, Dinner	1180	101	34	70
Chicken Scaloppine, Dinner	1410	68	42	112
Eggplant Parmesan, Dinner	1270	117	44	69
Fettuccine Alfredo	1220	71	28	93
Layers of Lasagna, Dinner	1110	82	69	59
Primo Chicken Parmesan, Dinner	1650	116	74	98
Spaghetti & Meat Sauce, Dinner	1120	83	42	69
Veal Marsala	1300	136	36	67
Veal Parmesan	1130	100	46	61
Chianti Steak	1290	74	79	74
Chicken Portobello	910	75	45	47

Food	Calories	Carb (g)	Protein (g)	Fat (g)
Pollo Margo "Skinny Chicken" **	320	29	41	5
Simple Salmon **	590	15	52	32
Pasta Milano, Dinner	1530	125	58	98
Penne Rustica, Dinner	1590	93	96	92
Seafood Linguine	1230	85	62	64
Lobster Ravioli	1350	101	48	84
Sicilian Four-Cheese Ravioli	1390	69	69	92
Margarita Pizza (whole pizza) *	1020	124	49	35
Sicilian Pizza	1460	125	73	72
Chocolate Tiramisu	1030	106	8	63
Italian Sorbetto w/ Biscotti	240	58	3	1
Smothered Chocolate Cake	1390	139	13	84

*Good choice
**Best choice

Fast Food Restaurant: McDonald's

Food	Calories	Carb (g)	Protein (g)	Fat (g)
Hamburger	250	31	12	9
Cheeseburger	300	33	15	12
Double Cheeseburger	440	34	25	23
Quarter Pounder w/cheese	510	40	29	26
Big Mac	540	45	25	29
Filet-O-Fish	380	38	15	18
McChicken	360	40	14	16
Premium Grilled Chicken Classic Sandwich *	420	51	32	10
Premium Crispy Chicken Classic Sandwich	530	59	28	20
Premium Grilled Chicken Ranch BLT Sandwich	470	53	36	12
Ranch Snack Wrap(Crispy)	340	33	14	17
Ranch Snack Wrap (Grilled) *	270	26	18	10
Honey Mustard Snack Wrap (Crispy)	330	34	14	16
Honey Mustard Snack Wrap (Grilled) *	260	27	18	9
Small French Fries	230	29	3	11

Food	Calories	Carb (g)	Protein (g)	Fat (g)
Med. French Fries	380	48	4	19
Large French Fries	500	63	6	25
Chicken Nuggets (6 piece)	280	16	14	17
Chicken Selects Premium Breast Strips (5pc)	660	39	38	40
Barbeque Sauce	50	12	0	0
Honey	50	12	0	0
Hot Mustard Sauce	60	9	1	2.5
Sweet 'N Sour Sauce	50	12	0	0
Spicy Buffalo Sauce *	70	1	0	7
Creamy Ranch Sauce	200	2	1	22
Tangy Honey Mustard Sauce	70	13	1	2.5
Premium Southwest Salad with Grilled Chicken **	320	30	30	9
Premium Southwest Salad with Crispy Chicken	430	38	26	20
Premium Asian Salad with Grilled Chicken **	300	23	32	10

Food	Calories	Carb (g)	Protein (g)	Fat (g)
Premium Asian Salad with Crispy Chicken	410	31	28	20
Premium Caesar Salad with Grilled Chicken **	220	12	30	6
Premium Caesar Salad with Crispy Chicken	330	20	26	17
Butter Garlic Croutons	60	10	2	1.5
Snack Size Fruit & Walnut Salad *	210	31	4	8
Newman's Own Creamy Southwest Dressing	100	11	1	6
Newman's Own Creamy Caesar Dressing	190	4	2	18
Newman's Own Low Fat Balsamic Vinaigrette **	40	4	0	3
Newman's Own Low Fat Family Recipe Italian Dressing **	60	8	1	2.5
Newman's Own Low Fat Sesame Ginger Dressing	90	15	1	2.5
Newman's Own Ranch Dressing	170	9	1	15
Egg McMuffin	300	30	18	12

Food	Calories	Carb (g)	Protein (g)	Fat (g)
Sausage McMuffin	370	29	14	22
Sausage McMuffin with Egg	450	30	21	27
English Muffin *	160	27	5	3
Bacon, Egg & Cheese Biscuit	430	37	16	24
Sausage Biscuit with Egg	510	36	18	33
Sausage Biscuit	430	34	11	27
Southern Style Chicken Biscuit	410	41	17	20
Biscuit	260	33	5	12
Bacon, Egg & Cheese McGriddles	420	48	16	19
Sausage, Egg & Cheese McGriddles	560	48	20	32
Sausage McGriddles	420	44	11	22
Big Breakfast	740	51	28	48
McSkillet Burrito with Steak	570	44	32	30
Hotcakes (w/o Syrup & Margarine)	350	60	8	9
Hotcakes and Sausage (w/o Syrup & Margarine)	520	61	15	24
Hotcake Syrup	180	45	0	0
Sausage Patty	170	1	7	15
Scrambled Eggs (2) *	170	1	15	11
Hash Brown	150	15	1	9

Food	Calories	Carb (g)	Protein (g)	Fat (g)
Fruit 'n Yogurt Parfait	160	31	4	2
Apple Dippers *	35	8	0	0
Low Fat Caramel Dip	70	15	0	0.5
Vanilla Reduced Fat Ice Cream Cone *	150	24	4	3.5
Kiddie Cone **	45	8	1	1
Strawberry Sundae	280	49	6	6
Hot Caramel Sundae	340	60	7	8
Hot Fudge Sundae	330	54	8	10
Peanuts (for Sundaes) **	45	2	2	3.5
McFlurry with M&M's Candies (12 fl oz cup)	620	96	14	20
Chocolate Triple Thick Shake (16 fl oz cup)	580	102	13	14
Baked Hot Apple Pie	250	32	2	13
Cinnamon Melts	460	66	6	19
McDonaldland Cookies	250	42	4	8
Chocolate Chip Cookie	160	21	2	8
Oatmeal Raisin Cookie	150	22	2	6
Sugar Cookie	160	21	2	7

Notes for McDonald's items:

*Good choice
**Best choice

Restaurant: PF Chang's

Food	Calories	Carbs (g)	Protein (g)	Fat (g)
Chang's Chicken Lettuce Wraps	377	35	28	12
Chang's Vegetarian Lettuce Wraps *	281	37	25	4
Seared Ahi Tuna **	210	9	26	9
Harvest Spring Rolls	287	30	6	15
Crab Wontons	440	32	19	26
Wonton Soup – Bowl	354	44	21	10
Chang's Chicken Noodle Soup – Bowl	512	30	64	13
Hot and Sour Soup - Bowl	652	82	37	18
Hot and Sour Soup – Cup **	85	11	5	2
Chicken Chopped Salad	401	21	47	14
With Our Signature Ginger Dressing add	483	9	1	48
Moo Goo Gai Pan	661	32	54	34
Lo Mein with Beef	1374	94	67	80

Food	Calories	Carbs (g)	Protein (g)	Fat (g)
Lo Mein with Shrimp	1134	97	43	64
Almond and Cashew Chicken	815	63	81	30
Beef with Broccoli	1118	38	93	65
Sweet and Sour Chicken	764	107	40	20
Chang's Spicy Chicken	923	88	56	37
Ginger Chicken with Broccoli	656	45	60	26
Kung Pao Chicken	1228	58	74	79
Sweet and Sour Pork	1095	106	61	46
Mu Shu Pork	871	50	57	50
Mongolian Beef	1178	29	96	73
Wild Alaskan Sockeye Salmon Steamed with Ginger	646	23	60	36
Cantonese Shrimp **	330	21	33	12
Oolong Marinated Sea Bass	521	40	64	12
Chang's Lemon Scallops	952	100	69	28

Food	Calories	Carbs (g)	Protein (g)	Fat (g)
Kung Pao Shrimp	977	58	60	58
Sichuan from the Sea Calamari	1078	118	69	36
Chow Mein with Beef	793	84	54	26
Chow Mein with Shrimp	625	84	41	13
Double-Pan Fried Noodles Combo	1384	118	68	69
P.F. Chang's Fried Rice with Chicken	1208	151	47	44
P.F. Chang's Fried Rice Combo	1539	154	68	69
Brown Rice – Cup	254	53	5	2
White Rice – Cup	295	64	6	1
Buddha's Feast - Steamed **	137	29	8	1
Buddha's Feast - Stir Fried	367	66	25	5
Shanghai Cucumbers **	124	8	10	6
Spinach Stir-Fried with Garlic – Small **	77	9	7	3

Food	Calories	Carbs (g)	Protein (g)	Fat (g)
Sichuan-Style Asparagus-Small **	97	16	6	3
Apple Pie Mini Dessert	170	34	1	4
Carrot Cake Mini Dessert	295	42	2	14
S'Mores Mini Dessert	323	50	3	12
The Great Wall of Chocolate Cake	2237	376	20	90
Stock Velveted *	- 150-300	- 29		- 15-30
Light or No Oil	- 150-250	- 29		- 15-25
Light Sauce, No Sauce or Sauce on the Side **				

-Uses vegetable stock instead of oil, giving dishes a lot less fat
-Less sodium and/or sugar
*Good choice
**Best choice

Restaurant: Starbucks

Drink	Calories	Carbs (g)	Sugar (g)	Protein (g)	Fat (g)
Skinny Latte (Caramel, Vanilla, Hazelnut, or Cinnamon Dolce)	130	19	17	12	0
White Hot Chocolate	490	63	62	16	19
Signature Hot Chocolate	470	57	46	15	24
Tazo Chai Tea Latte	240	44	41	7	4
Strawberries & Crème Frappuccino	570	95	83	12	15
Double Chocolaty Chip Frappuccino	510	78	59	14	19
Caramel /Mocha Frappuccino Light Blended Coffee	160	30	21	5	1.5
Caramel Frappuccino	380	57	48	6	15
Cappuccino	120	12	10	8	4

Drink	Calories	Carbs (g)	Sugar (g)	Protein (g)	Fat (g)
Iced Brewed Coffee	90	21	20	0	0
Iced Caffe Mocha	320	38	28	9	17

*Values are for Grande size drink made with 2% milk.

Fast Food Restaurant: Subway

Food	Protein (g)	Carbs (g)	Fat (g)	Calories
6" ham sandwich *	18	47	5	290
6" oven roasted chicken breast *	24	47	5	330
6" roast beef sandwich *	19	45	5	290
6" subway club sandwich *	24	47	6	320
6" sweet onion chicken teriyaki *	26	59	5	370
6" turkey breast sandwich *	18	46	4.5	280
6" turkey breast and ham sandwich *	20	47	5	290
6" veggie delite sandwich	9	44	3	230
6" cold cut combo (cold)	21	47	17	410

Food	Protein (g)	Carbs (g)	Fat (g)	Calories
6" tuna (cold) sandwich	22	45	31	530
Ham Deli *	11	36	4	210
Roast Beef Deli *	13	35	4.5	220
Tuna Deli	14	35	18	350
Turkey Breast Deli *	13	36	3.5	210
6" toasted cheese steak	24	47	10	360
6" toasted chicken & bacon ranch	36	47	25	530
6" toasted chicken parmesan	26	64	18	510
6" toasted chipotle southwest cheese	24	48	20	450
6" toasted Italian BMT	23	47	21	450
6" toasted meatball marinara	24	63	24	560
6" toasted spicy Italian	21	46	25	480

Food	Protein (g)	Carbs (g)	Fat (g)	Calories
6" toasted subway melt	25	48	12	380
chicken & bacon ranch	41	18	27	440
Tuna wrap	27	16	32	440
Turkey & bacon melt	31	20	24	380
Turkey breast wrap **	24	18	6	190

All sandwiches include standard vegetables

*Good choice (high carbs, but lower fat)

**Best choice (lower carb and fat)

APPENDIX 3

ANATOMY CHARTS

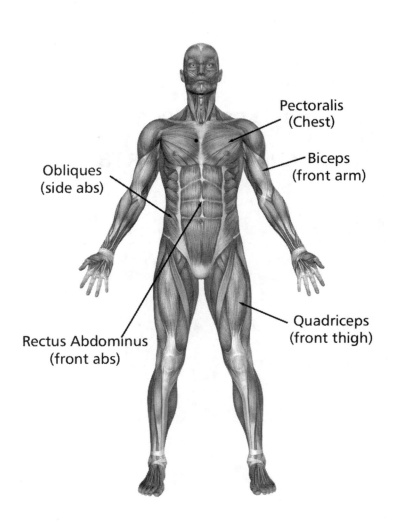

Pectoralis
(Chest)

Biceps
(front arm)

Obliques
(side abs)

Quadriceps
(front thigh)

Rectus Abdominus
(front abs)

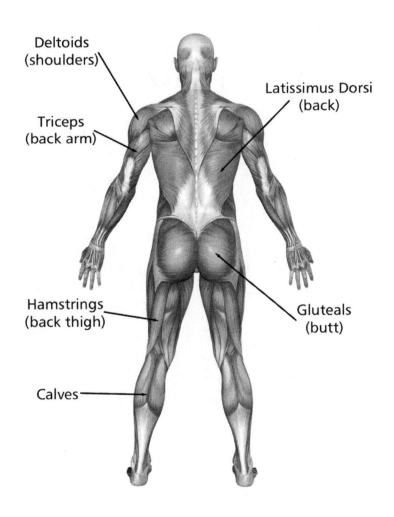

Deltoids
(shoulders)

Triceps
(back arm)

Latissimus Dorsi
(back)

Hamstrings
(back thigh)

Gluteals
(butt)

Calves

APPENDIX 4
FOOD LOG

FOOD LOG

Date: _____

Breakfast	
AM Snack	
Lunch	
PM Snack	
Dinner	
Other Foods	
Exercise (Type & Duration)	

INDEX

ABOUT THE AUTHOR

Anu Morgan was born in India in 1975 and moved to the United States at age two. She grew up in Glendale Heights, Illinois, a suburb of Chicago, and later attended the University of Illinois where she was awarded a B.S. in Biology in 1997. She presently lives and works in Houston with her husband, Scott, and their two children, Jasmine, age four, and Jaiden, age three. She initially worked as a weight loss consultant with a major national weight loss center. In 1999 she began her career as an ACE certified personal trainer and has been helping Houston area clients achieve their weight loss and fitness goals ever since.

GET REAL ABOUT WEIGHT LOSS
ONLINE RESOURCES

www.GetRealAboutWeightLoss.com – This site is all about this book and how to follow the Get Real plan and reach your weight loss goals. It contains a great deal of information and resources on weight loss. You can also subscribe to Anu's free online newsletter to get the latest tips and ideas on how to get and stay in great shape.

www.GetRealZone.com – This is Anu's private membership site. Highly recommended for anyone serious about losing weight or maintaining their level of fitness. And for a limited time you can get a **one month free trial membership**.

www.AnuMorgan.com - Anu's blog that contains links to all the Get Real resources and products.

www.BodyFitHouston.com Anu's website for her Houston area personal trainer business.

A Special Offer For You

Hi, this is Anu Morgan with one last message – I really want you to achieve your weight loss goal and the best way to make that happen is for you to have resources, support, and accountability. I know that not everyone can afford a personal trainer. That is why I created GetRealZone.com, my private membership site. It provides you with everything you need to reach all your fitness goals. GetRealZone.com gives you:

- online videos with detailed instruction for all of the exercises and stretches shown in this book, and many, many supplemental exercises
- a monthly teleseminar with me on weight loss, nutrition, and many other subjects directly related to helping you achieve your weight loss goals
- a library of articles on weight loss related topics
- a membership forum where you can post questions and connect with other people who are on the same journey as you
- healthy recipes
- and a whole lot more

The best part is that if you act now you will receive a FREE month membership in GetRealZone.com.

Just go to GetRealZone.com and click on the **"JOIN NOW"** button on the homepage to get started now!! I am excited for you and I wish you all the best!

Anu Morgan